THE FOOT & ANKLE SOURCEBOOK

The Foot & Ankle Sourcebook

EVERYTHING YOU NEED TO KNOW

M. David Tremaine, M.D., and
Elias M. Awad, Ph.D.

LOWELL HOUSE
Los Angeles

CONTEMPORARY BOOKS
Chicago

Library of Congress Cataloging-in-Publication Data

Tremaine, M. David and Elias M. Awad
    The foot & ankle sourcebook : everything you need to know / M. David
Tremaine and Elias M. Awad.
        p. cm.
    Includes Index
    ISBN 1-56565-438-2
    1. Foot—Care and hygiene. 2. Foot—Diseases. 3. Ankle—Wounds and injuries.
I. Tremaine, M. David. II. Title. III. Title: Foot and ankle sourcebook.
RD563.A97
617.5'85—dc20   94-23247
                                                  CIP

Lowell House books can be purchased at special discounts when ordered in bulk for premiums and special sales. Contact Department JH at the address below.

Publisher: Jack Artenstein
General Manager, Lowell House Adult: Bud Sperry
Text Design: Nancy Freeborn
Illustrations: Sean Cliver

Manufactured in the United States of America
10 9 8 7 6 5 4 3 2 1

This book is dedicated to Ann Tremaine, without whose help this project would not have come to fruition. With love and appreciation.

Acknowledgments

The authors wish to acknowledge a number of people whose contributions made this book possible.

We are indebted to Rima D. Irani, P.T., HealthSouth Of Arlington, Virginia and G. Elizabeth McKenna, M.P.T., A.T.C., Skyline Physical Therapy and Sports Medicine Center, Arlington, Virginia, for producing the initial draft of Chapter 16 on Physical Therapy and Rehabilitation.

We especially thank Drs. Jung Kim, Staff Anesthesiologist, National Hospital For Orthopaedics and Rehabilitation, Arlington, Virginia, for providing professional help in preparing Chapter 17: "Your Foot Surgery and Anesthesia"; Dr. Joseph H. Kaufman, Dermatologist, Alexandria, Virginia, for his invaluable review of Chapter 13 on the dermatological problems of the foot; Dr. Virgil Balint, Chief Of Physiatry, National Hospital For Orthopaedics and Rehabilitation, for significant contribution to Chapter 14: "Industry/Occupational Foot Problems."

We wish to thank National Hospital Medical Center in Arlington, Virginia, for its support of the treatment of foot and ankle diseases and disorders.

We owe a great deal to the team of professionals at RGA Lowell House who have been models of talent. We salute our editor, Bud Sperry, who provided timely motivation and invaluable support. Special thanks to Maria Magallanes, managing editor, who coordinated and helped with the preproduction of the manuscript.

Table of Contents

Preface

In today's fast-paced world, health care has become an important political, social, and economic issue. People in general are becoming more concerned with their well-being than ever before. With educational media, the average citizen is gaining more knowledge about health care and preventive medicine. This type of literacy makes it easier to work with and treat patients. In fact, the recovery process can also be affected.

The focus of this book is on "THE FOOT & ANKLE"—a guide to the detection, maintenance, and management of the many aspects of the human foot. In the book, we emphasize the causes, treatment, rehabilitation, and prevention of foot problems. It is a useful source for the whole family, people with existing foot problems, the ten million people with diabetic foot problems, senior citizens with geriatric feet, the work force with work-related injuries, and as an educational tool.

Why this book? There are a number of reasons that prompted us to write this book:

- There are foot problems in all age groups. The lay person needs basic knowledge about the foot and ankle to assist him in decision making. They often come for a medical consultation when self-help from this book would be a viable option. This sourcebook can be a useful money-saver.

- Long before a person becomes a patient, an up-to-date guide to the human foot is invaluable for self-help, awareness, and preventive maintenance which could otherwise result in costly work time lost, suffering, and unnecessary expense. People also want to know about their feet for fear of becoming prematurely immobile. Every time there is a potential foot problem, patients have been known to develop psychological and traumatic problems fearing they could lose the ability to walk.

- In sports, the foot is of prime importance. At home, on the road, and in sports, 30 to 40 percent of people develop ankle sprains with persisting problems after they heal. A number of basic steps and preventive measures prescribed in this book are timely, cost-saving, and contribute to the proper maintenance and health of the lay person's foot.

- The problems of diabetic foot disease have been known to account for a significant percentage of a $15 billion industry. Diabetic foot problems are the third leading reason for hospital admissions. For example, a patient who stepped on a nail resulted in an infected foot, prolonged hospitalization, loss of three toes, and a $50,000 hospital bill. The goal of this book is to significantly lower disabling diabetic foot problems and minimize the chance of amputations which are traumatic to most patients.

- In today's mass production of cheaper and ill-fitting shoes, more and more people suffer from foot problems. In a recent Women's Shoe Survey, for example, eighty-eight percent of the respondents reported one foot bigger than the shoe, and over eighty percent of those with such a problem reported pain or deformity.

- People in general want to know how to use metatarsal and other pads, and advice on self-help for various foot problems resulting from ill-fitting shoes, etc. This book addresses these and other problems. There is also a solid chapter on bunions, hammer toes, corns, and calluses, and when they should be treated. In this book, we dispel many myths about foot care and explain in easy-to-understand language the causes of and how to treat the most common foot ailments.

We have witnessed over the years a profound increase in medical knowledge. Unfortunately, limited attention has been given to the foot for today's layman. The foot continues to be an overlooked appendage of the body until it begins to show signs of wear, tear, pain, or immobility. With the limited number of books on the subject, we believe this book is a timely contribution to the layman.

We feel that this is a highly readable and fast-paced book about foot and ankle problems and diseases. There is no medical jargon to confuse the reader. It is more like bringing medicine of the foot to the level of the layman. It is an easy to follow, step-by-step, explanation of function, cause, treatment, and management of the foot. Each chapter ends with a summary ("In a Nutshell"), terms to remember, and "doctor's corner," addressing key foot and ankle problems and how they were treated.

For detailed medical discussion of foot and ankle problems and deformities, the following books are recommended:

- Jahss, Melvin H., *Disorders of the Foot and Ankle: Medical and Surgical Management* (2nd ed.) Philadelphia, Penn.: W. B. Saunders, 1991.

- Levin, Marvin E. and O'Neal, Lawrence W. (eds.), *The Diabetic Foot* (4th ed.) St. Louis, Mo.: Mosby Company, 1988.

- Mann, Roger A. and Coughlin, Michael, *Surgery of the Foot and Ankle,* vol. 1 (6th ed.). St. Louis, Mo.: Mosby Company, 1993.

- Techdjian, Mihran O., *Pediatric Orthopedics.* Philadelphia, Penn.: W. B. Saunders, 1991.

M. David Tremaine, M.D   Elias M. Awad, Ph.D

PART I

~

Overview

CHAPTER 1

Oh, My Aching Feet

INTRODUCTION

Welcome to this user guide to the human foot. Feet are among the most neglected and abused part of the human anatomy. It has been known for years that foot problems are associated with medical ailments such as diabetes, arthritis, and gout. In fact, almost 90 percent of Americans experience pains and discomfort with their feet. According to the National Center for Health Statistics, 10 percent of all Americans and 25 percent of the elderly have serious foot problems. Yet, over 75 percent of them do not seek professional help.

We all know the punishment our feet go through every day. With each step we take, our feet cushion a force of up to three times our total body weight. Over thirty million Americans run or jog every day and millions more participate in other sports such as aerobic dancing, sports, biking, and walking. Our feet work hard to carry us over hard surfaces , up and downhill, and on uneven terrain.

Feet take on our daily stresses and strains. When they hurt, we hurt all over. They are often cramped into ill-fitting shoes which frequently cause corns, bunions, and painful problems in the back and elsewhere in the body. Yet amazingly the feet that make us mobile are the most neglected and taken for granted parts of the body. We falsely believe that foot pain comes naturally from age, taking part in sports, or our occupations.

Our hardworking feet are the "wheels" and the shock absorbers of the body. From the hip down, they are a complex system. They consist of bones, joints, tendons, ligaments, muscles, blood vessels, and nerves designed to adapt and flex with virtually any uneven surface, terrain, or weight change. Combined with the knees, legs, hips, and back, they work together in amazing fashion. Think of the car you drive and the many parts that make it possible for this vehicle to transport you everywhere. Yet all it takes is one part to fail or show signs of wear, and the whole system may break down. In our "foot system", any breakdown can cause pain, irritation, and degradation in the quality of life.

Foot problems are partly hereditary and partly caused by structural deviations. Experts disagree as to the relative contributions of one or the other. For example, some experts estimate that ninety percent of bunions are hereditary; others attribute foot problems to footwear that can cause bunions, calluses, hammertoes, and tendinitis, as well as back and hip pain. In shoeless societies, there are few painful bunions or hammertoes. There is no question that shoes which are too small, too narrow, or too short compel a redistribution of body weight and force a change in how a person walks. This often leads to muscle and ligament problems of the lower legs and eventually to serious foot deformities.

Athletes as well as lay people experience footwear problems. How many times have you heard someone recommending one brand or type of shoe over others? How often do you wear one type of shoe for one type of activity? How do you know whether you need lightweight versus sturdy shoes for your sport? What should the soles be made of? What about the lining? Many sports professionals have trouble matching their activities and their foot structure with their shoes. As a result, foot problems develop.

Your occupation and overall lifestyle also enter the picture. They give you clues to your foot problems. Salesmen, nurses, store clerks, bar-

John, a twenty-five year old teacher, arrived at a clinic with severe pain and thickened calluses on the ball of his foot. He had a very high arch and tight heel cord (achilles tendon). His medical history revealed he had been treated for this problem at age six by soft arch supports to relieve the pressure under the ball of the foot. He continued to have problems and tried a variety of supports, therapy, and anti-inflammatory medicines. By then his foot was quite rigid and hard to fit with shoes. His activities were becoming increasingly restricted. He elected a surgical procedure, triple arthrodesis, to fuse or stiffen the foot, and to release ligaments to allow a better weight bearing foot. Simpler or less complex surgery at an earlier age, before the growth plates fused and when soft tissues were more pliable, might have been a better option.

At present, John is almost back to normal function, but he is likely to develop arthritis in other joints in the future. Losing foot flexibility transfers stresses to other joints of the foot and lower extremities.

Identifying and appropriately treating a medical problem at an early age may alleviate more serious and significant problems later in life.

tenders, and teachers wear different kinds of shoes than construction workers, truck drivers, and mail carriers. Their occupations require more walking and standing which causes foot stress and strain. This needs to be accommodated with appropriate shoes. Keep in mind that some foot pain is more easily tolerated than others and requires little treatment. Significant pain requires immediate treatment. In any case, wearing comfortable shoes with plenty of toe room and exercising regularly are the first basic rules to minimizing discomfort due to calluses and bunions.

One indication of increasing foot problems is the steady surge in the number of orthopedic surgeons and podiatrists. Women form the majority of patients and undergo most of the operations for bunions and hammertoes. Foot surgery is not a minor procedure and is not a guaranteed cure. For example, researchers have reported a twenty to thirty percent recurrence rate after bunion surgery. Surgery also means restricting your activities for an extended time period. Some incisions heal in a matter of weeks; for others, including bone remodeling, the healing can take months. Given the age, physical condition, and occupation of the patient, postsurgical complications should also be considered.

In addition to hereditary and footwear problems, the popular drive to be physically fit has focused close attention on foot problems. Over 50 percent of American adults participate in one form of exercise daily. Thirty-five million Americans play tennis, and twenty-six million swim at least three times each week.

The key questions asked by physically active people are: What is the safest sport? How can I prevent injuries? How fast do I heal? Will running make ankles and knees arthritic? Do all broken bones heal?

USER GUIDE

Help is in this guide. It is designed to bring you the facts, explain foot problems, and discuss complicated diseases and medical decisions in layman's language. I will tell you when you should see a doctor because of persistent foot and ankle pain, joint injuries, or loss of function. I also explain length of recovery from injuries like a broken toe, a sprained ankle, or muscle, joint, ligament, or tendon problems.

One important inclusion in this book is a section on the diabetic foot. Over fifteen percent of diabetics develop foot ulcers, primarily because of repetitive stress to insensitive feet. Of the diabetics, twenty percent who are admitted to the hospital have foot problems and thirty percent have peripheral vascular disease. Approximately six out of every thousand diabetic patients undergo amputation. The hospital cost for amputations in the U.S. is probably over $3 billion annually, not including rehabilitation, lost income, or lost jobs. Obviously, the goal is to prevent this tragedy.

I want to caution you that no book can be a cure–all, or a replacement for the medical professional. There are also many aspects of the foot that are not fully understood. Recent advances in orthopedics provide hope for more and more patients to get relief from foot pain. Many of these advances include sophisticated imaging techniques using computers to provide patients with an accurate and reliable treatment program to prevent long-term problems. There is also computerized gait analysis (a study of how we walk and run) which has given us better insight into stresses that can cause foot problems such as bunions, hammertoes, and pinched nerves or neuromas. Also, recent advances in surgical techniques have made it possible to treat certain foot problems with a greater degree of precision and at much less risk or discomfort to the patient. These details are also covered in this book.

HOW THE BOOK IS ORGANIZED

The foot approach traces foot and ankle problems that can begin in childhood, continue through adulthood, and persist into old age. There are conditions that apply to all ages, with varying times of onset and degree of severity. We have only one pair of feet for our lifetime, so let us learn how to take care of them.

The book is divided into five major sections for ease of use. Each section consists of several chapters with the following format:

- **Introduction**—what the chapter offers.

- **Symptoms/case studies.**

- **Natural history**—progression.

- **Treatment**—nonsurgical, surgical, and rehabilitation.

- **Prevention, answers to common questions, and helpful hints.**

- **Terms to remember**—these terms are also included in the glossary at the end of the book.

Part I is an overview of the foot, its structure, and function. Chapter 1 discusses the importance of the foot and ankle and how their health can affect your lifestyle. Chapter 2 emphasizes the basic anatomy of the foot and ankle and their interrelationships to other parts of the body. The second part of the chapter refers to functions of the various parts of the foot and ankle and explains how different movements during walking, like pronation and supination, can affect your gait.

Part II deals with foot and ankle problems that occur as birth problems or during childhood. Chapter 3 discusses the common childhood problem of turned in feet, and handles early identification of other common foot problems such as high arches and flat feet. These are dealt with in detail in the adult section. Chapter 4 deals with congenital deformities, such as club feet, that appear in infants.

Part III focuses on adult foot and ankle problems. Chapter 5 deals with bunions, small toe bunions (bunionettes), hammertoes, mallet toes, and claw toes. Chapter 6 deals with troublesome afflictions such as metatarsalgia, calluses, corns, warts, ingrown toenails, and athlete's foot. Chapter 7 addresses nerve problems such as neuromas. Chapter 8 focuses on common heel pain problems. Chapters 9 and 10 discuss flat feet and high arches.

Part IV covers general diseases or injuries affecting the feet that are common to all ages. These include diabetes, arthritis, common sports injuries and fractures, and general foot problems. In chapter 10, we cover the general diabetic problem associated with the foot. Chapter 11 deals with arthritis and how it might turn into a serious problem for your feet. Chapter 12 discusses sports injuries like tendinitis, stress fractures, sprains, and so on. It also deals with the trauma of ankle fractures, dislocations, and broken foot bones. Chapter 13 tackles nail and skin problems. Chapter 14 deals with industry/occupational foot problems. Chapter 15 addresses the important question, "Am I wearing the right kind of shoes?" The chapter talks about shoes, orthotics, and braces. In chapter 16, we talk about physical therapy and rehabilitation—exercises or rehabilitation programs for foot and ankle sufferers. Finally, chapter 17 is a guide to surgery and anesthesia.

Part V is composed of the last chapter (18) which is a section in itself. It addresses old-age (geriatric) foot problems—what to look for in the way of foot and ankle problems related to senior citizens.

At the end of the book, you will find a glossary of important terms, a list of common foot agencies and related associations, a glossary of medical specialists in the foot and ankle area, and a list of associations and support groups.

HOW TO USE THIS BOOK

This book can be used in a number of ways. For one, if you have a specific problem, you may turn to the appropriate chapter. For example, if you have sores from ill-fitting shoes, you may want to refer to chapter 15, or to related material in chapter 5 on bunions, or in chapter 6, on corns and calluses. If you have children with specific problems, chapter 3 would be the place to start. There are also problems that afflict children and adults alike, where other chapters might be of use to you.

You may also use this book to learn about different treatments of foot and ankle problems. This means starting from the beginning and continuing through the material as you see fit. The material is fast-paced and easy to read. We have varied each chapter to include photographs of ailments, art sketches, and case situations to illustrate selected areas of concern.

A third way to use this book is by section. For example, if you're interested in children's problems, then Part II would be the one to focus on; for adult foot and ankle problems, read Part III (chapters 5-9). Regardless of the approach you take, each chapter ends in a section called "In a Nutshell," which is more of a super-summary—questions and answers typical of what patients ask their doctors, and select terms to remember. These improve your vocabulary, so the next time you talk with your doctor you should begin to understand some terms. The glossary at the end of the book is a comprehensive compilation of the terms used in the foot and ankle specialty.

CHAPTER 2

What Do I Need to Know About My Feet?

INTRODUCTION

Humans rely on their feet to take them everywhere. Healthy feet are always ready, whether you want to walk, swim, hike, dance, run, or simply stand still. Your feet take an endless beating and log an average of 1,000 miles each year. As shock absorbers, they cushion millions of pounds of pressure during one hour of strenuous exercise. For example, during a one-mile run, your feet carry a total weight of up to five tons.

When even one foot begins to hurt or is injured, a person feels somewhat vulnerable, because it is more difficult to walk and get around. It is important, then, that you understand the anatomy of the foot, its importance to the body, and how to keep it healthy.

All parts of the foot must work together for a healthy posture and function or a combination of problems can develop.

BASIC ANATOMY

Your foot is a small but complex unit. The basic anatomy of the foot consists of:

- twenty-eight bones—thirty-two joints covered with cartilage
- ligaments
- muscles/tendons
- nerves
- blood vessels/blood circulation
- skin and soft tissues.

See figure 2-1.

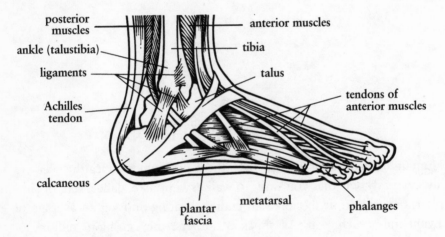

FIGURE 2-1. *Bones, joints, ligaments, and muscles of the foot*

FUNCTIONAL ANATOMY

All the foot parts work together as a unit and are integrated into the rest of the body to help you perform a variety of body movements and weight bearing chores. Remember the old song, "the foot bone's connected to the knee bone, the knee bone's connected to the hip bone, . . . the hip bone's connected to the back bone . . . " This brings up the important relationship of the foot and ankle to the body. See figure 2-2.

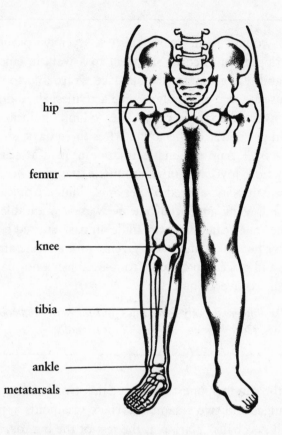

hip

femur

knee

tibia

ankle
metatarsals

FIGURE 2-2. *Anatomy relationship: foot, knee, hip*

Frequently, abnormalities in distant joints or bones will cause referred symptoms in the foot or vice versa. Examples are arthritis, tendinitis, ligament strains, and fractures. We are fortunate that our body allows the foot to adapt to uneven terrain, changing its mode with every step.

Functional Segments

There are four functional segments of the foot complex: Forefoot, mid-foot, hindfoot, and heel. See figure 2-3.

The Forefoot

The **forefoot** (ball and toes of the foot) serves primarily as a platform for propulsion. Also called the anterior foot, the forefoot has five toes (**pha-langes**) and five long bones (**metatarsals**) with associated joints. The big

J oyce, a woman in her early thirties, severely sprained her ankle tripping on a curb. She went to a walk-in emergency center and was given an Ace bandage wrap, told to rest her ankle, use ice, and gradually resume activities. She didn't have crutches and favored her ankle, causing her to limp significantly. She felt she would get better on her own. After three days, she experienced severe back pain and made an appointment at our clinic. Upon examination, Joyce had obvious muscle spasms in her back—a result of her gait being altered by her ankle injury. Ironically, her ankle was some-what improved but she was very disabled with back pain. She was treated with an ankle air cast, started on physical therapy for her ankle and back, given pain medicine and muscle relaxants, and placed on crutches to re-establish a normal walking pattern. She recovered quickly.

Note: *A limp is abnormal body mechanics and may trigger problems in many other areas. Crutches may be your "best friend."*

toe (**hallux**) is the number one toe. It contains two smaller toe bones called the phalanges and two sesamoids. These sesamoids appear on x-ray as two small "eyeballs" staring at the rest of the big toe. The other toes each contain three phalanges and two joints (**interphalangeal joints.**) Additional joints (**metatarsal phalangeal joints**) provide the important rollover capability at the ball of the foot.

The Midfoot

The midfoot has five short bones and the main arch. They act to stabilize and support body weight like a set of ball bearings or shock absorbers. These midfoot bones are linked to the hindfoot and forefoot by small intrinsic foot muscles and the important arch ligament (**plantar fascia**).

The Hindfoot

This part of the foot links the ankle joint to the midfoot. The *talus* is the central bone making up this complex of three joints. The ankle joint is composed of the top of the talus and the end of the two leg bones (**tibia and fibula**). This hinge joint allows you to move your foot up and down.

Subtalar Joint.

The heel (**calcaneus**) is the largest bone in the foot. Its bottom surface is covered with a layer of fat forming a heel cushion. The joint between the talus and the heel is the subtalar joint. The talus also forms a joint with the navicular bone and the calcaneus with the **cuboid**. This complex of three joints is called the *triple joint.*

The midfoot and hindfoot operate together in order to absorb shock, walk on uneven surfaces, and push off properly. Their combined motion is called either pronation or supination.

FIGURE 2-3. *Parts of the foot*

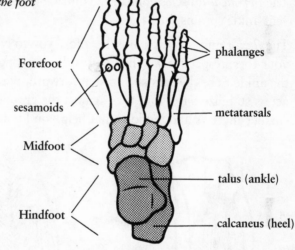

Forefoot

phalanges

sesamoids

metatarsals

Midfoot

talus (ankle)

Hindfoot

calcaneus (heel)

MUSCLES, TENDONS, AND LIGAMENTS

As you can see, bones and joints are critical to proper foot functioning, but they simply cannot survive the day-to-day routine without the support of muscle, tendon units, and ligaments.

Muscles produce movement by contracting or pulling on their connected tendons which move the bones and joints. *Tendons* are elastic structures connected to the fleshy muscle. These tendons may become overstressed, ruptured, or inflamed (**tendinitis**). Every muscle that contracts has the capability to relax. For example, the calf muscles (gastrocnemius and soleus) and their common tendon (**Achilles tendon**) have a joint function that makes it possible to run, jump, rise on your toes, or walk upstairs. The Achilles tendon is the strongest and best known tendon in the body. Athletes and others who exercise regularly know the tendon well, because it is commonly injured.

There are other muscles to consider:

- The *anterior tibial* muscle allows you to move your foot up toward your shin.

- The *posterior tibial* muscle supports the arch.

- The *peroneal* muscles control the outside of the ankle to help prevent ankle sprains.

- The *flexor* and *extensor* muscles allow you to bend and straighten your toes, respectively. When you walk, the long extensors help the ankle raise the toes and to step forward, while the long flexors act as stabilizers for your toes against the ground. There are also smaller muscles and tendons that help you lift and curl your toes.

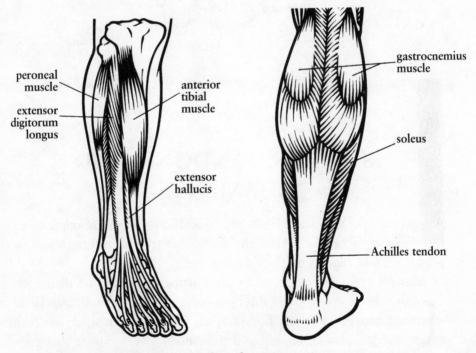

FIGURE 2-4. *Muscles of the leg: posterior and anterior*

N ick, an active 50-plus recreational tennis player, lunged to the net to get a drop shot—then felt like his calf had exploded and thought someone had kicked the back of his leg. He was helped off the court. At his clinic examination, an indentation was felt at the site of his Achilles tendon. There was bruising (ecchymosis) around the injury, and Nick was unable to stand on his toes or point them downward.

The treatment Nick elected was to surgically repair the rupture. Nick wore a short leg cast for eight weeks and continued physical therapy for an additional two months. He was gradually able to resume his recreational tennis in six months.

Ligaments are tissue fibers that connect bones together to stabilize joints. The longest ligament in the foot, called *plantar fascia*, runs along the sole as shown in figure 2-5. When you are standing, this ligament stretches from the heel to the toe and the arch flattens. This provides balance and comfort. As you raise your heel, the plantar fascia tightens to help form the curvature of the arch. It provides a strong foot for push off.

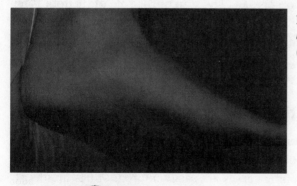

FIGURE 2-5. *Plantar fascia by exam—shortened arch (contracted)*

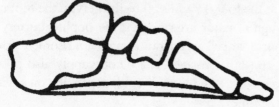

Plantar fascia extended (foot lengthened)

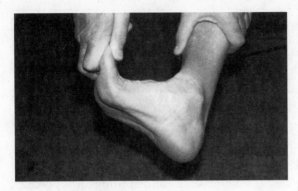

FIGURE 2-5. *Plantar fascia by exam—shortened arch contracted*

Plantar fascia contracted (foot shortened)

The Skin

The skin is the largest organ of the body. The vascular inner skin (dermis) regenerates surface cells to preserve the quality, smoothness, and general condition of the outer skin. The skin of the sole of the foot is ten times as thick as that of the rest of the human body. Its purpose is to withstand the punishment feet take each day. Yet, such a durable skin is vulnerable to all kinds of problems such as corns, calluses, blisters, infections (athlete's foot or warts), and pressure ulcers.

The Nerves and Blood Supply

Muscle function and skin sensation is made possible by nerves. The nerves that go to the foot are cordlike fibers that originate in the lower part of the spinal cord. Some nerves are easily injured; others are deeply embedded and protected in the foot. In addition to the nerves, the foot is supplied with blood through a major artery called the **popliteal artery**. Blood is an important source of cell regeneration and nourishment for the bones, muscles, skin, and other tissues. The blood supply also promotes circulation which keeps the foot warm or cold, depending on environmental conditions at the time.

THE DYNAMIC ANATOMY—THE FOOT DURING WALKING

It is important to understand how the parts of the foot help you walk and run. The sequence of movement used in walking and running is called the *gait cycle*. It is heel strike to heel strike. When you are standing, the heel outside (lateral side) of the midfoot and the forefoot bear even weight distribution. The arch ligament (plantar fascia) supports the midfoot arch. This should be a relaxed, comfortable position.

When you walk, the body weight strikes the ground at the outer back part of the heel. The heel pad cushions the heel at impact. The heel strike is the beginning of the *stance* (weight bearing) phase. Then the weight moves along the outer edges toward the ball of the foot and all the way to the big toe. The foot sags slightly in the arch—a motion called *pronation*. Pronation is necessary for the foot to absorb the impact of the body weight. See figure 2-6.

Once the foot is solidly on the ground, it begins to move in the opposite direction of pronation. First, the heel rises and the foot lifts up and out, rising on the toes or ball of the foot. This acts like a lever to propel the body forward. The brunt of the work is borne by the big toe, as it encounters the pressure first. Then the thigh extends and lifts the body up

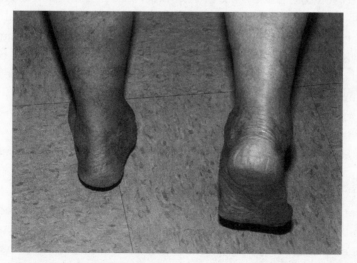

FIGURE 2-6. *Pronation (left foot), supination (right foot)*

and forward, putting the foot through the heeloff-toeoff-pushoff phase. It is during this three-phase cycle that supination occurs.

Stability is provided by *supination* and is the stiff foot phase of walking. It is the rolling outward of the foot. The back ligament (plantar fascia) tightens during this push off phase. When you push off to walk, the stress is on the ball of the foot. Much of this stress is absorbed by the big toe. In extreme supination, picture getting off a horse and standing in a bowlegged position that extends all the way down to the outside of the foot.

You can now understand how commonly such pressures on the foot can lead to injuries and potential deformities. Weight is a major factor in foot problems and injuries. Overweight people are more likely to have foot problems later in life than people with average or below average weight. But regardless of weight, factors such as the types of exercise you do, your age, the shoes you wear, and your occupation all have something to do with the potential health or status of your foot.

Normal gait progresses from pronation to supination in a smooth and almost automatic fashion. Very few people think about or worry about how they walk, unless they have obvious problems. The bones, muscles, joints, thighs, legs, and back all work together to make sure this fascinating mode of "transportation" is to your liking.

Each individual's gait is unique. Just stand on a street corner and watch how people walk. Some walk briskly, others seem to amble. Also keep in mind the many factors that affect the gait cycle, including physical, structural, and emotional. Physically, excessive pronation forces an unnecessary twisting of the foot and extra pressure on the heel, arch, and big toe. Instead of bouncing back, the pronated foot tends to sag and appears flat and limp. This causes uneven weight distribution, which means one part of the foot is taking on extra baggage. Muscles enter the picture trying to compensate for the difference, resulting in muscle strain. Overpronated feet often cause or contribute to the formation of bunions, hammertoes, bursitis, calluses, joint injuries, or even pain in the neck and upper back.

Although excessive pronation is a more common source of foot problems, other people tend to oversupinate, which is demonstrated by a pigeon-toed gait and thickened calluses along the entire outer foot surface. The tendons and joints strain because the foot is more rigid and less shock absorbing, and a propensity for ankle sprains are common complications.

Women tend to overpronate more than men because they have loos-er joints and more flexible ligaments and tendons in the feet. With ath-letes, it can be devastating. Women also have a tendency to oversupinate, causing a pigeon-toed gait. This means the toes point inward during walking, which can be inefficient and painful. It can also cause tendon and ankle strains. Again, athletes find oversupination a nuisance.

IN A NUTSHELL

It is important to know the functional anatomy of your foot. From the hip bone to the foot bone, your foot parts have to work togeth-er as an integrated unit for proper functioning. It is necessary for your midfoot and hindfoot to operate together for proper pronation and supination. The normal gait cycle includes both motions in an automatic fashion.

It is worth remembering that your bones and joints cannot survive the day-to-day routine without the support of muscles, tendons, and ligaments. The skin, nerves, and blood supply also play a major role in ensuring healthy feet. The important point to keep in mind is never to take this marvelous "transportation system" for granted. It requires care and maintenance, especially as you grow older.

TERMS TO REMEMBER

Achilles tendon: The heel cord which is an extension of the calf muscle and controls the ability to rise on the toes; a large tendon located in the back of the ankle.

Ankle joint: Top of the talus and the end of the two leg bones of the foot.

Calcaneous: Heel of the foot; the largest bone in the foot.

Extensor muscle: A muscle that allows you to straighten your toes.

Fibula: The smaller of the two bones between the ankle and the knee.

Flexor muscle: A muscle that allows you to bend your toes toward the floor.

Forefoot: Ball and toes of the foot; anterior foot.

Gait cycle: The sequence of movements in walking and running, including heel strike to push off.

Hallux: The big toe.

Ligament: Additional supportive tissue fibers holding two joint bones together to stabilize them.

Metatarsal: One of five long bones of the forefoot.

Metatarsal phalangeal (MTP) joint: The joint at the end of each toe close to the web space associated with the ball of the foot.

Phalanges: A general term for small bones in the toes and fingers.

Plantar fascia: The longest ligament in the foot; the main arch ligament that connects the heel to the toes and runs along the arch of the foot.

Pronation: The rolling over to the inside of the foot while weight bearing. Overpronation flattens the arch and causes the toes to point out. Some pronation is normal during walking.

Stance: Weight bearing phase of walking.

Subtaler joint: The joint between the ankle bone and heel bone.

Supination: The rolling of the foot to the outside when weight bearing. Oversupination causes a pigeon-toed gait.

Talus: The ankle bone.

Tendon: Elastic structure connected to the fleshy muscle.

Tendinitis: Inflamed tendon.

Tibia: The larger of the two bones between the knee and the ankle.

PART II

Foot and Ankle Problems During Childhood and Adolescence

CHAPTER 3

What Should I Do About My Child's Turned-in Feet?

INTRODUCTION

A number of books have been written about foot deformities related to children. When it comes to foot problems, children suffer the same as adults. In fact, many foot problems that are left untreated could return to haunt them in adulthood. So it is important to discuss some of the most common children's foot problems (what they are, their causes, and treatment) and how parents should handle them.

Some foot problems go back to the positioning of the fetus in the uterus. The genetic basis of many foot problems also plays a role. The saying, "the apple falls very close to the tree," shows it is not uncommon

Concerned parents should ensure that there is no bony deformity in their children's hip, knees, or feet. Treatment should be considered if there is a family history of significant persisting angular deformities.

to see children with a variety of foot problems similar to those of their parents. In any case, there isn't much that parents can do about prevention other than to address the problem as soon as it is detected. With today's diagnostic and treatment procedures, children with foot problems can be treated effectively before more serious damage occurs.

Here is a parent's lament that we hear often:

"My child's feet turn in and he stumbles a lot. He seems to be awkward for his age. My pediatrician says he will outgrow this, but I'm concerned something is being missed!"

Fortunately, most in-toeing is a growth and development problem that will correct itself with little or no medical treatment. The important point to remember is to give your children's feet a close look—how they walk, what they say bothers them, and so on—and check with your doctor accordingly. With the knowledge and technology available today, there is no need for a child to be left without proper foot and leg care. Many common foot problems, if recognized early, can respond to conservative treatment.

The foot problems that you should be concerned about include:

• Club foot

• Metatarsus adductus

• Toe-in or toe-out (also called *femoral or tibial torsion*) of the hip and leg (usually not a problem)

• Bunions, flat feet, high arches, and leg length problems.

NATURAL HISTORY

When discussing your child's foot problem, a general understanding of how the leg and foot develop should first be clarified. This type of background may help relieve many of your parental anxieties. A child's first living environment is the uterus. This is a cramped condition for the baby as he or she reaches full term. In this environment, as growth and development is rapidly occurring, the legs are usually curled in or out and early body molding is taking place. Therefore, a variety of foot positions are present at birth. After birth, the foot looks relatively straight, is flexible, and moves easily. However, it appears flat. Much of this appearance is due to the excess of body fat and underdevelopment of the foot arch supporting muscles. See figure 3-1.

During the child's early development and walking phase (from about their first month until about age 2½), the arch begins to develop from muscle use. In this phase, restrictive shoes are discouraged because they only delay normal muscle development. In these early years, the entire foot often turns in and the knee caps may point to the inside instead of

Bow legs
(infant–2½)

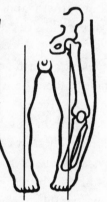

Normal
(Age 2½–3+)

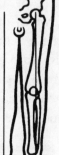

Knock knees
(Age 3–5+)

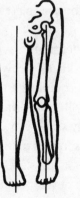

Normal
(Age 6+)

FIGURE 3-1. *Stages in the development of the legs*

straight ahead. The legs appear bow-legged because of the normal shape of the leg bones.

Bowing exists in most children, but luckily corrects itself once walking activities and coordination develop. By ages three to four, a reverse knock-knee appearance occurs, which usually adjusts to the more accepted moderately straight leg by age six. A plumbline drawn down the leg of your child will demonstrate this normal sequence from bowleg to knock-knee to straight leg. The knock-kneed posture causes pressure on the inside of the foot and your child's foot is naturally flatter during this growth stage.

Over ninety percent of bowleg or knock-kneed postures do NOT require treatment and should NOT be treated. If these conditions are severe, medical evaluation to rule out growth abnormality should be done. Your pediatrician can follow your child's development and watch for any severe deformity.

Not all bony foot structures are present at birth and some foot structures are soft cartilage in the early stage of life. These cartilage structures change to bone in a specific time sequence (years) during childhood to adolescence development stage. Foot growth in length is very rapid during the first year of life and then progressively slows down until age five. For girls ages five to twelve and boys ages five to fourteen, the average growth length is .9 centimeters (one-third-inch) per year. However, foot growth and bony maturation vary considerably as they do in other parts of the body. Diet, a variety of stresses that include high level competitive sports like gymnastics, and various illnesses may delay or alter this growth. Actual foot growth may not be complete in some individuals until age twenty or twenty-one.

Naturally, leg length is growing concurrently with the foot. Almost two-thirds of leg growth occurs at the knees' growth plates. The ankle and hip joint contribute the remaining growth. If a discrepancy in one of these growth centers occurs, one leg will be a different length than the other. It is understandable that the body's fine-tuned growth "machine" sometimes gets out of sync and one leg is longer than the other. Up to one-half-inch difference in leg length does not translate into symptoms if the difference is part of normal growth and development. A young child has the ability to alter growth and compensate dramatically for these leg length differences.

In contrast, a leg length difference of as little as one-quarter- to one-half-inch, caused by injury and occurring in late adolescence or adulthood, may cause symptoms. Some of these are backaches, knee pain, or even excessive pronation of one foot (usually the longer leg). This is a complex interplay which can best be evaluated by a specialist. A tip-off to leg length difference is an uneven waist, shoulder, or hem line. Occasionally, a noticeable curvature of the spine (**scoliosis**) or even an uneven gait will show up. These symptoms need to be evaluated as soon as possible.

With this basic information about foot development, we should discuss the more common developmental variations that are in-toeing from the hip or leg. Fortunately, these problems are usually outgrown or can be adjusted to with no known problems in over ninety percent of the cases as skeletal maturity is reached.

HIP AND LEG TORSION

Hip Torsion

Torsion is twisting of the leg and foot inward or outward, and hips or legs that turn inward or outward more than normal. *In-toeing* in children is understandably a common concern for you as a parent. This problem usually originates in the hip (femoral) or the leg (tibia). The whole leg may be turned in or turned out due to in-utero positioning.

As we stated earlier, during the child's early walking years (eighteen months to four years), the entire foot often turns in and the knee caps can point to the inside instead of straight ahead. In most cases, your child's deformity will gradually correct itself. The stress on the legs and feet from day-to-day activities brings the feet and knees forward, decreasing the in-toeing. With some children, however, either the feet or the knee caps straighten out, not both. Even if there is a slight in-turn, in the majority of cases it should not limit activities in any way. In fact, many of the fastest athletes have some in-turning of their feet or legs. Speed and performance is actually improved, as the in-turned foot is quite stable and strong. It also means strong push off and acceleration.

Leg Torsion

Leg or tibial torsion is a case where the child's knee cap points straight ahead, but the leg bones are twisted inward causing in-turning of the child's feet.

In terms of self-help treatment, not much is needed. I recommend positioning the young child in the crib while he or she sleeps or when he or she is sitting. A tincture of time and a normal growth and development cycle correct most leg torsion problems. Stretching exercises are usually recommended by your pediatrician.

With respect to medical or orthopedic treatment for leg torsion, sometimes night splints (Dennis Brown splints and bar) or shoes with the heels held together and the feet pointed outward may speed up developmental adjustments of this problem. For mild deformities, no treatment is necessary.

Although torsion problems are the most common childhood extremity problem, other serious and abnormal conditions which cause turned-in or turned-out feet should be considered. Congenital dislocated or maldeveloped hips are two such problems and require aggressive early treatment. Deformity from trauma or deficiency should also be evaluated. Treatment for these other conditions is frequently required and is individualized, depending on the diagnosis.

Parents should be cautioned that surgery before age nine to ten is rarely considered. As in hip torsion, if the in-leg turning is severe and functionally limits the child, osteotomy of the leg bone may be necessary at this age.

Self-Help Treatment

If you notice your child has in-turning or abnormal posture, the first person to contact is your pediatrician. Most pediatricians are well-attuned to growth and development problems and can advise you on the proper treatment. Meantime, changing your child's position while he is sleeping helps change the stress on his or her legs. Placing a rolled towel or sheet behind the baby's back will hold him on his side, preventing rolling over. Do not apply constricting shoes before your child walks, as they tend to restrict normal foot and muscle development.

Remember, it takes patience and understanding to deal with this problem. Overanxiety and overtreatment should be avoided as much as possible.

Medical and Surgical Treatment

How can you tell your child has hip torsion? Hip torsion is diagnosed by observing that the child's knee caps point inward and there is significantly more internal than external rotation of his or her hip. See figure 3-2. Long leg braces, twisting cables, and even casts have been used to treat hip torsion in children, but they are ineffective and sometimes harmful because they can stretch out normal structures. No treatment from the onset of the problem up to ages nine to eleven has been found to be effective or necessary. In adolescence, some knee cap instability or foot strain may occur. Knee bracing and leg exercises or foot orthotics may be needed at this time.

Once again, natural growth and development will take care of most of these children's torsion problems. From ages nine to eleven, if the hip torsion causes the child to remain awkward and his hip out-turning is

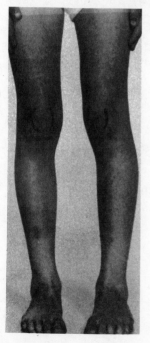

still significantly restricting, a surgical correction (osteotomy or bone realignment) of the femur (thigh bone) may be necessary.

FIGURE 3-2. *Femoral torsion: hip turns in.*
Note: kneecap points inward

J. T., a concerned mother, brought her three-year-old daughter to my foot-and-ankle clinic. The child had been walking since age eighteen months with a pigeon-toed gait. Mom was concerned that the toddler appeared clumsy, tripping and falling easily. Her pediatrician had advised her not to worry and just to perform some stretching exercises with the child. My examination revealed that the toddler's knee caps pointed inward and her feet pointed towards each other, as well. Her gait was awkward and hip torsion was suspected because of her inward pointing knee caps. Her hips showed double the normal in-turning motion. Normal hips are usually about equal between in-turning and out-turning, but this can vary greatly in the early walking years. In the past, bracing was used but provided little success. My advice to the mother was to let growth and development correct the problem for the next few years. Her pediatrician continued to watch the child, as well. I saw the little girl again at age eight, and found her to have normal, straight feet and only slightly in-pointing knee caps. Her clumsiness had disappeared and she had a normal gait.

In conclusion, a concerned parent would be advised to consider the following:

- Ensure that there is no bony deformity in your child's hips, knees, or feet.

- If there is a family history of significant, persistent angular deformities, treatment may be necessary.

- If developmental torsion or normal developmental bow legs or knock knees is the correct diagnosis, then minimal if any medical treatment is necessary.

IN A NUTSHELL

Most in-toeing problems in early childhood are development problems that will correct themselves without medical treatment. A child's bones have the ability to model and adapt to compensate for leg length differences, torsion problems, knock-knees, bowlegs, and other minor problems. Your pediatrician will pay attention to these developmental stages and will monitor your child's growth. More serious problems such as congenital dislocated hips, club feet, metatarsus adductus, or deformed feet need early medical treatment, however.

DOCTOR'S CORNER: QUESTIONS AND ANSWERS

My four-year old daughter has been diagnosed as having internal tibial torsion. No treatment was recommended. Should she be wearing any foot or leg braces?

The diagnosis of internal tibial torsion versus internal femoral torsion needs to be correctly determined first. There is no evidence to support wearing braces for internal femoral torsion, and it may even be harmful. For internal tibial torsion problems, however, some physicians feel that leg or foot braces worn for a few years help children remodel faster and better. Others disagree and feel that a child's natural growth and development will handle and correct the problem.

My three-and-one-half-year-old son is knock-kneed and looks clumsy, but he is quite active. Should I be worried about his condition?

Your pediatrician is no doubt watching your son's development and at this point he is in a "normal" stage of knock-knees that many little children go through. Most kids outgrow this condition without any medical intervention. As in other growth and development conditions, there is a wide range of "normal appearances" and most need no treatment. They will adjust themselves with growth. Casting and bracing have not proven helpful.

TERMS TO REMEMBER

Bowleg (genu varum): The knees are spread apart while the ankles and feet are close together. It may or may not be associated with additional torsion problems.

Congenital dislocated hips: A birth defect of abnormal hip joints where the ball is dislocated from the socket. It requires early identification and treatment for best results.

Femur: The thigh bone with the top end making up part of the hip joint.

Internal femoral torsion: In-turning of the entire leg including the hips and thighs. The knee caps point inward.

Knock-knee (genu valgum): The knees are touching or close together and the feet are spread apart. It may or may not be associated with additional torsion problems.

Pigeon-toed turning feet: It may be related to internal femoral torsion, internal tibial torsion, or both.

Scoliosis: A noticeable curvature of the spine.

Tibia: The larger of the two bones between the knee and the ankle.

Torsion: Twisting of the leg and foot inward or outward.

CHAPTER 4

Common Childhood Defects: Club Foot, Metatarsus Adductus, High Arches

INTRODUCTION

In this chapter, we want to talk about two of the most common abnormal toeing-in problems experienced in children which should be distinguished from the more common torsion problems. These are the *club foot* and *metatarsus adductus* deformities. In addition, the *high arch* or *cavus* problem is discussed. This condition is usually identified as a problem during childhood.

> Club foot and metatarsus adductus are the most common abnormal toeing-in problems experienced in children. Correcting the child's deformity while still maintaining his or her foot flexibility is critical.

CLUB FOOT

The club foot is probably the most significant congenital fixed deformity of the foot. Found more commonly in boys than girls, the club foot has a genetic tendency and is considered a defect of prenatal development, or is related to the cessation of normal foot development.

Natural History

Club foot deformity occurs at birth and can involve one or both feet. The foot may be flexible or very rigid. By rigid, we mean it cannot be straightened when examined. Unfortunately, the deformity affects the entire foot which makes it both dysfunctional and painful. The forefoot is rotated with the sole pointing inward. All toes are also turned inward rather than straight ahead and the heel is angled inward (inverted) as well. The whole foot points downward and the heel cord is also tight. See figure 4-1.

Self-Help Treatment

Club foot treatment should be initiated quickly after birth. Cursory self help such as massage, corrective shoes, or passive exercise only delays proper treatment and could decrease the chances of easy correction. You simply need to seek medical help from an orthopedist right away.

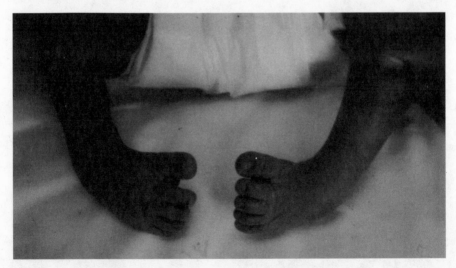

FIGURE 4-1. *Club foot*

Medical Treatment

Manipulation, stretching, casting, bracing, and taping are instituted with babies even while they are still in the nursery. When the foot is flexible, at least initially, full correction is possible but may take months. These techniques must be done correctly and meticulously under the supervision and guidance of an orthopedic surgeon. After the correction is obtained, further casting in the overcorrected position is done for three to six more weeks. Afterwards, night splints and manipulative stretching for ten to fifteen minutes four or five times a day are recommended. The child should wear shoes with special straight lasts or tarsal pronation shoes (outside heel and sole wedges). This treatment should be continued until normal walking and normal shoe wear patterns have been ensured. This could mean several special shoe changes.

Surgical Treatment

Surgery is the next step when the deformity is not correctable by other means or when certain parts of club foot deformity recur, causing abnormal pressures. Surgical correction is being performed at an increasingly early age, but not before three months at the earliest when the foot structure has formed adequately. When early surgery is done, only the tight ligaments require release as the child has the ability to remodel his own foot.

Later surgery in a six- to eight-year-old requires bony realignments (**osteotomies**). This type of surgery secures a better weight-bearing foot. The foot may not be a totally normal looking foot, but function is the main goal. If correction is not made until after the foot is fully grown (usually ages ten to eleven), fusion or stiffening of the hindfoot joints in the corrected position may be necessary. *Fusion* is a surgical procedure where extra bone is used to provide a fixed joint in order to secure a more stable position.

In terms of surgical expectations and complications, good results have a lot to do with how correctable and flexible the foot was at the beginning of treatment. On the average, the earlier the surgery, the more flexible and normal the foot will become. The stiffened foot means prolonged treatment and surgery and may still have residual stiffness. Because of this stiffness, more stress is placed on the other foot joints which may result in arthritis in these joints later in life. The thing to remember is early treatment of club foot deformity, as it gives the best and most lasting results.

METATARSUS ADDUCTUS (SKEW FOOT)

This problem is a common condition in newborn infants and is a congenital deformity. It involves the forefoot, but not the heel. It is sometimes called a third of a club foot. The toes of the foot point inward but are not rotated. Frequently, the big toe points inward more than the other toes. See figure 4-2. This is not a severe deformity, although children may walk in an awkward manner and often trip over their own feet. They also wear out shoes early and the wear pattern is distorted.

Natural History

The incidence of metatarsus adductus is about 1 in 1,000 births and is slightly more common in girls than boys. The deformity also seems to run in families and is ten times more common than club foot. This condition can be adequately corrected, but correction without adequate follow-up leads to failure.

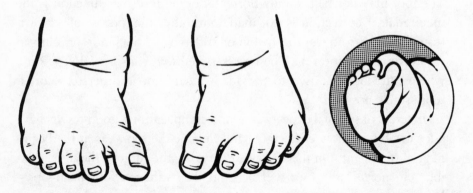

FIGURE 4-2. *Metatarsus Adductus*

Self-Help Treatment

If the adductus deformity is recognized, evaluation and treatment by an orthopedic surgeon is recommended as soon as possible. Home stretching, if done improperly, can be detrimental and should not be started without proper instructions. The case history below demonstrates that if the child is treated early enough, preferably by age three, stretching exercises may be the only treatment necessary.

Medical Treatment

Treatment should begin early. Properly performed stretching exercises are recommended right away. If the foot is not correcting, taping or casting in the nursery, or even a few months to a year later, can correct the problem. Reverse last shoes for pronators do *not* help. In fact, they may make the problem worse. After casting or other corrections have been done, night casts are frequently used. Night casts are removable casts worn at night to correct heel pain and other foot problems.

J ohnnie, a two-year-old, was brought to my office by his parents. He had been walking for over six months, displaying in-turned feet. His parents had accepted this as natural clumsiness from learning to walk. Some months later, his feet still turned in.

After examining the toddler, I found his hips and knees to be in a normal position. However, the front of his feet were significantly curved inward. He had metatarsal adductus. I treated him with a series of casts to stretch out his feet, more with each cast change.

After three months of casting, Johnnie's feet were straight. No more casts were applied and his feet were further protected by wearing straight last* shoes. His parents were instructed in proper stretching techniques to be performed several times a day. The child continues to progress normally.

*A last is the form over which a shoe is constructed

Surgical Treatment

Surgery may be recommended at any time after age one or two if significant persisting deformity or functional problems exist. It requires the evaluation of an experienced orthopedic surgeon to predict the severity of the deformity. Like club foot surgery, early surgery only requires surgical release of ligaments. After about age six, club foot or metatarsus adductus surgery requires bone correction. Later in life, people with metatarsus adductus may develop troublesome bunions, flat feet, or be displeased with the cosmetic appearance of their feet.

Even when only milder forms of the metatarsus adductus exist, these secondary problems may need to be addressed when they develop. The approach and treatment of these is discussed and individualized in the subsequent chapter. In terms of expectations and results, the expectations for metatarsus adductus are better than for club feet.

HIGH ARCH (PES CAVUS)

The saying, "No two feet are alike" is true, but there are those that are far enough from the norm that their deviation can be spotted by an experienced naked eye. One of the common features of an abnormal-looking foot is the high arch or cavus foot. High arch is a difficult problem to deal with. Although its symptoms may not be noticeable until adulthood, occasionally a stiff high arch will be diagnosed and require treatment during the development years.

Natural History

The high-arched foot is a worse shock absorber than the normal arch. Its shape puts undue pressure on the metatarsal heads of the foot when the forefoot is bearing weight. People with high arches often develop symptoms at an early age. When the high-arch appearance is obvious, it may be associated with some neuromuscular disease causing imbalance. This can be muscle disease or dystrophy, spinal or other nerve problems, polio or myelomeningocele (spine deformity), cerebral palsy, or Charcot Marie Tooth disease.

The natural history of the deformity depends upon the diagnosis. Almost one-fourth of high arch problems are classified as idiopathic (meaning the cause is unknown). Associated problems are:

- Claw toes or hammertoes with calluses
- Metatarsalgia
- Arch pain—heel pain
- Recurrent sprained ankles

Medical Treatment

It is very important to do diagnostic tests to identify the underlying cause of high arch problems. We also need to take a careful family history and rely on examination to look for associated neuromuscular diseases. For example, x-rays of the spine, nerve electrical and muscle electrical studies, electromyograms (EMG), nerve conduction velocities (NCV) tests, and occasionally a MRI or Myelogram are all important. Appropriate treatment follows, depending on the diagnosis. In the meantime, proper shoes for cushioning are helpful. Metatarsal pads or molded shock absorbing orthotics may help relieve the symptoms of high-arch feet.

Stretching of the heel cord and plantar fascia after proper physical therapy instruction is also important and should be performed daily. Even small gains in flexibility may substantially improve the shock absorbing function of the foot.

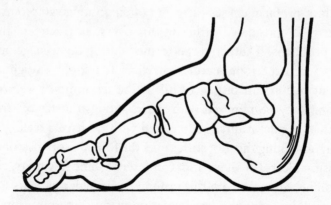

FIGURE 4-3. *High arch or cavus foot*

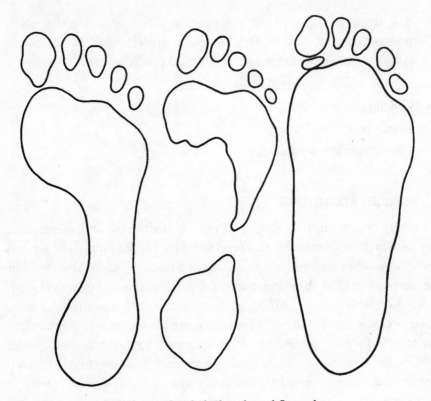

FIGURE 4-4. *Footprints of normal arch, high arch, and flat arch*

Surgical Treatment

This rigid foot problem causes early and often limiting symptoms. As a result, surgery is considered earlier in this course of treatment than in other foot problems. If surgery is performed during the teenage or early adult years when the foot is still somewhat adaptable, realigning the foot without fusion can be successful. If the deformity is very established, fusion may be required with the resulting transfer of stress to other joints. If the deformity is associated with decreased feeling in the foot, fusion or making the foot stiffer puts the foot at more risk of developing pressure ulcers. In an attempt to preserve some flexibility, corrective osteotomies are used with this group even in older patients.

In any case, knowing the serious nature of this deformity can make early treatment important.

IN A NUTSHELL

Congenital foot deformities generally need early orthopedic treatment and often even surgery. The goals are to correct the child's deformity while still maintaining the flexibility of his or her feet. Treatment that is done late due to recurrence of the deformity or failure of treatment requires more extensive bone realignment or even fusion procedures. The older the child is when corrective surgery is done, the more lasting foot stiffness he or she will suffer.

High arches tend to cause shock-absorbing problems and metatarsalgia even at an early age. It is important that an appropriate medical evaluation be done to look for underlying causes of the problem. Modifications of lifestyle, including less impact-type sports, shock absorbing foot wear, and even bone realignments may be needed. Ligament release may be required at a relatively young age.

DOCTOR'S CORNER: QUESTIONS AND ANSWERS

My eight-month-old baby has club feet. He has been treated with casts and now my orthopedist has recommended surgery. Isn't he too young for an operation?

With improved techniques such as the usage of an operating microscope, effective surgery can be performed on patients at an early age. Experience has taught us that the earlier the club foot deformity is corrected and the sooner the ligaments are released, the more flexible and permanently corrected the foot will be. Usually, this club foot surgery is done between the ages of six months and one year, depending on the surgeon's training, experience, and professional opinion.

My fifteen-year-old son has high arches and toes that seem to curl up. Should he try to stretch out his arches and toes? What else should we do?

In contrast to flat feet, extremely high arches often are associated with some underlying neurological problem. Clawing toes with high arches are even more significant. Your son needs to have a complete medical workup to identify any possible nerve or muscle problem. A common diagnosis could be Charcot Marie Tooth disease which is usually hereditary and has varying degrees of severity and different rates of progression.

It is important to have a complete and accurate diagnosis for a treatment plan, as well as genetic counseling. It is also important to identify any loss of sensation on the bottom of your son's feet that could coexist with his high arches. If there is a loss of sensation, he is a candidate for foot ulcers.

After his medical evaluation, even if no symptoms are present, I would recommend that he get good shock-absorbing shoes and do a daily stretching program. This won't change his arch, but it will help him gain as much arch and toe flexibility as possible. If he is athletic, I would encourage low-impact sports for him.

TERMS TO REMEMBER

Cavus foot: A foot with a high arch.

Club foot (talipes equinovarus): In this birth defect, the heel cord, ankle, arch ligament, and joint are extremely contractive (tight), causing the toes and heels to point down and inwards. The forefoot (metatarsal) bones are also pointing abnormally inward.

Fusion: A surgical procedure in which extra bone is used to provide a fixed joint in order to secure a more stable position.

High arch (pes cavus): See cavus foot.

Last: The form over which a shoe is constructed.

Magnetic resonance imaging (MRI): A diagnostic procedure using a complex magnet, radio waves, and atomic nuclei. It is an excellent study to show soft tissue problems (ligaments, tendons, blood vessels).

Metatarsalgia: A painful condition, usually on the ball of the foot.

Metatarsus Adductus (Skew foot): A foot deformity that involves the forefoot and not the heel; front part of the foot turns inward at birth. It needs early correction with exercise and sometimes casting or surgery.

MRI: See magnetic resonance imaging.

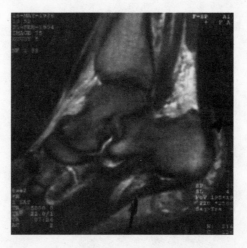

FIGURE 4-5. *MRI. Arrows point to the Achilles tendon and arch ligament (plantar fascia).*

Night cast: A removable cast worn at night to help stretch the heel cord and eliminate heel pain.

Osteotomies: Realignment of the foot; realignment bone correction.

Skew foot: See Metatarsus Adductus.

PART III

Adult Foot and Ankle Problems

CHAPTER 5

What Can I Do About My Bunions and Toe Pain?

There was a young lady of Crete
Who was so exceedingly neat,
When she got out of bed
She stood on her head
To make sure of not soiling her feet

—BENNETT CERF, *Out On a Limerick*

Most foot problems involve the forefoot. They include problems with the big toe bunion, hammertoes, mallet toes, small toe bunion (bunionette), and/or neuromas.

INTRODUCTION

If your feet could "think," they would probably scheme to revolt. Fortunately, they cannot do anything beyond voicing their complaints through the language of pain. Foot problems like bunions, bunionettes, mallet toes, hammertoes, and claw nails are the most common foot problems. Most of these problems are preceded by early symptoms that are easily spotted. These subjects are discussed in order to provide you with a clear understanding of these troublesome deformities and the best approach to take in dealing with them.

WHAT IS A BUNION?

For centuries, humans have been plagued by bunions—a small swelling, a bump, an abnormality, or a deviation in the big toe joint. A bunion is not a skin disorder or a tumor. Many people believe that once they have a bunion, the only treatment they are stuck with is surgery. Bunions are a very common problem. They generally do not require surgical intervention and many of them do not hurt.

A bunion is a big toe that is misaligned at the joint and results in an unsightly bump. The ligaments are stretched out and the tendons which move the big toe pull it farther out of line. They become a deforming force and often cause the bunion to worsen. This is a gradual process occurring over many years, and makes comfortable shoes difficult to find.

The anatomy of a bunion is shown in figure 5-1. The metatarsal head is pushed medially (toward the midline of the body). *Metatarsal* is one of five long bones of the forefoot. In addition, the phalanx (small bone of the big toe) begins to point toward the second toe. The end of the metatarsal may become quite enlarged. Pressure from the big toe can also lead to deformity in the second toe, causing it to point toward the third toe. The second toe may lay on top of the big toe or beneath it.

Bunions can be quite painful. Pain may be due to bursitis (inflammation in the soft tissue over the bunion bump). There may also be referred pain in the metatarsal pad with associated calluses in this area. This pain is caused by the second toe having to bear additional weight that is normally supported by the first toe.

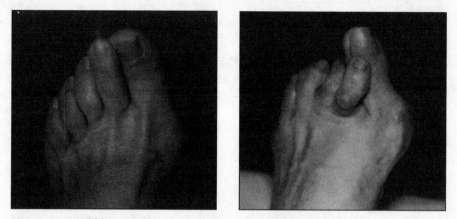

FIGURE 5-1. *Mild bunion (left) severe bunion and hammer toe (right)*

What Causes a Bunion?

There is truth to the fact that bunions appear more frequently in certain families than in others. The shape of your foot is genetically inherited. This means you may have a certain susceptibility to foot deformities like bunions. Yet, other lucky members of the family may never develop this problem.

Bunions frequently occur in people with flat feet and in those having medical conditions such as rheumatoid arthritis, gout, and neuropathies. Bunions may occasionally develop after traumatic injuries. In those societies where no shoes are worn, bunions rarely exist and when they do, are painless. Wearing shoes that are too narrow or narrow shoes with high heels have caused a high incidence of painful bunions in women.

A recent study shows that in childhood girls have twice as many bunions as boys. In the military population, women have triple the bunion problems. In the adult surgical census, women requiring bunion surgery outnumber men as much as 15 to 1. Properly fitting shoes are your best defense in relieving pressure from bunions and other toe deformities. There is no question that tight shoes are *hazardous* for your feet.

Natural History

Bunions that begin in childhood and are symptomatic (hurt) very likely will become worse later in life. Some bunions gradually develop arthritis in the big toe. Most bunions continue to increase their angle of deformity and cause pressure, pain, and calluses at some point. However, some fortunate folks with bunions won't get arthritis and their bunions don't seem to worsen. There are other bunions that are not painful as such, but over time produce symptoms in other toes or nails. In any case, bunions are a nuisance and often cause shoe fitting problems. They may involve both feet, with one foot usually more symptomatic and deformed than the other.

Symptoms

You usually begin to notice your bunion when you feel pressure against your shoe. As the angle of the bunion gets worse, it begins to push against adjacent toes. When this happens, several symptoms begin to get your attention:

- toes start to overlap.
- ingrown toenails form.
- nerves between the toes become irritated (neuromas).
- a hammertoe forms on the second or third toe.
- painful calluses develop under the second or third toe.
- the big toe loses most of its function of weight bearing and abnormal pressures transfer to the outside of the foot.
- A callus forms near the tip of the big toe because it is rotated abnormally. See figure 5-2 for a photo of a bunion and callus.

Self-Help Treatment

A recent Hong Kong study showed that bunions were endured by 33 percent of the business population, while shoeless boat people living on sampans appeared to have no bunion problems. The best favor you can do for yourself is to wear *extra depth shoes* that have a *wide toe box*. See chapter 15 for information about proper shoe-fitting techniques.

Another helpful hint is to stretch shoes at the bunion point at a shoe repair shop. Moleskin "doughnuts" or pieces of tubefoam over the bunion bump may also help relieve pressure. These aids are usually available over the counter. If you have a bunion and tight heel cords (Achilles

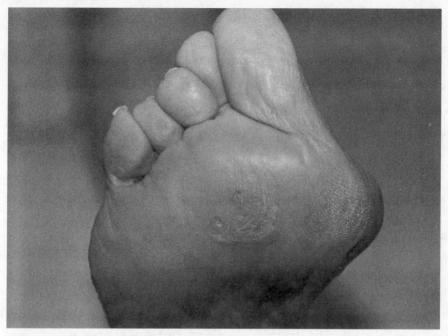

FIGURE 5-2. *Bunion, calluses under metatarsal heads*

tendon), you may benefit from daily heel cord stretching and foot strengthening exercises.

A number of other devices may help the bunion problem:

- Over-the-counter arch supports can help take the pressure off your big toe, especially if you have flat feet.
- Soft spacers like tube foam or lamb's wool placed between your toes may also relieve bunion pain and pressure.
- Metatarsal pads placed in shoes behind calluses have been known to relieve pressure and make you more comfortable.
- Ice packs used on the painful area several times a day may reduce swelling and inflammation.

None of these will hurt you and, indeed, may help reduce your painful bunion symptoms.

Medical Treatment

Patients seek treatment of bunions for cosmetic reasons as well as for pain. Bunion treatment is individualized and depends on the age of the patient, the nature of the deformity, and the severity of the symptoms attributed to the bunion. If the patient is under twenty years of age, chances are the bunion is related to family history. In this case, the treatment is to wear a shoe that corrects pronation. Sometimes a stabilizing splint is worn at night or a shoe may be cut out at the site of the bunion. In the elderly, bunions are normally treated by wearing molded or extra depth, wide toe box shoes that prevent pressure on the protruding portion of the foot. Exercise and corrective shoes should always be considered before surgical intervention.

A number of non-steroidal anti-inflammatories (NSAIDs) like ibuprofen (Motrin, Advil, Indocin, and so on) or aspirin may help reduce the inflammation and swelling in your big toe caused by bunions. Occasionally, bunions are associated with gout which is an acute inflammatory process with elevated blood or joint fluids containing uric acid crystals. This very painful condition is sometimes triggered by life stress or surgical stress. Its treatment requires medical evaluation and is often dramatically relieved by medicines like indocin.

Most over-the-counter or prescribed medicines have potential side effects. Non-steroidal anti-inflammatories may cause stomach problems and should be taken after you have eaten. If any side effect symptoms appear, you should stop taking the medicine and call your doctor. Prolonged use of such medicine requires monitoring by your doctor.

You may benefit from professionally fabricated orthotics which can help take pressure off painful bunions, especially if you have flat feet. Custom fabricated shoes may be needed if you have a deformed foot, especially if you also have a medical condition like rheumatoid arthritis or diabetes.

You may get relief from your bunion pain by getting an injection using cortisone and an anesthetic like Xylocaine. These injections are used sparingly.

G loria, a middle-aged attorney, came to our clinic with complaints of mild, aching pain and redness over her great toe bump. Her shoes were uncomfortable, causing pain, especially at the end of the day.

Upon examination and x-rays, I found a prominent bunion on her left great toe. There was inflammation and redness present, and the pain increased when I pressed on it. Her great toe motion was normal and painless, but she had a painful callus under her second toe metatarsal pad. Her shoes were high heels with pointed toe boxes. They were also one-half-inch narrower than the ball of her foot.

Initial treatment included a change of shoe to extra depth sport shoes with a wide toe box. These were to be worn to and from work, and she changed to lower heeled, wider dress shoes for her business meetings and more formal occasions. A metatarsal pad was placed in her shoe to relieve pressure on the callus.

What Gloria sacrificed in fashion, she gained in comfort and function. So far, she has not required any other treatment for her bunion.

Surgical Treatment

Medical literature cites more than one hundred surgical procedures for correcting bunion deformities. In the past, surgeons chose a procedure based more on their training than the type of deformity involved. Better understanding of foot mechanics and research over the past ten years has helped base the choice of type of surgery on the cause of the patient's bunion deformity. Tight ligament structures are released surgically, while loose capsule ligaments are tightened. Tendons are frequently shifted to create a better pulling angle (known as modified McBride procedure.)

Most surgical bunion procedures require bone surgery as well. The enlarged bony bump on the big toe is removed and the metatarsal bone is cut (osteotomized) to straighten the toe and narrow the foot. Frequently, surgical pins, screws, plates, or wires are used to provide necessary stability to the bone. These are usually left in the foot and are not rejected by the body. Pins that protrude through the skin are easily removed in the doctor's office after healing has taken place.

When your bunion deformity is severe, and/or there is painful arthritis associated with it, just straightening your toe will not be an adequate solution. Remember, bunions that do not have arthritis do not hurt when you bend your toe. Their pain is caused by abnormal pressures. Arthritis pain is joint pain and will even be felt when you are not wearing your shoes. The surgical treatment for this problem is either fusion (arthrodesis) of the great toe in a straight position, replacement of the joint with an artificial device, or removing one half of the joint (Keller procedure).

All of these methods have been successful in relieving the arthritis pain, but sacrifice of the joint is necessary. Fusion is usually the correct choice, especially if you are active and put a lot of stress on your toe. Despite the fact that the bones are fused, there is no limp associated with arthrodesis and it is 90 percent successful in relieving pain. In most cases when this procedure is used, the toe is already very stiff and has acted as a partly-fused toe for years. The artificial joints used are mechanical devices (machines). In contrast to the outstanding results obtained with total knee and total hip replacements, the toe artificial joints tend to fail mechanically rather quickly. At this time, there are no long-term studies documenting prolonged success. However, work continues to be done to improve these devices.

Sometimes, severe secondary problems like recurring ingrown toenails or painful calluses, hammertoes, or mallet toes are caused by bunions and require surgery. The bunion will need surgical correction as well, even though the bunion itself may not be painful.

When Should I Have Bunion Surgery?

The main points to consider in your decision should be:

- Bunion pain that is unrelieved by proper shoes.
- Progressive toe deformity.
- Inability to fit into reasonable shoes.

There may also be severe secondary problems caused by the bunion that interferes with your lifestyle. In any case, just remember that, by itself, the unattractive cosmetic appearance of the foot is a limited reason to suggest bunion surgery. Surgery, per se, can be serious for a variety of reasons.

Surgical Expectations

Bunion surgery is usually performed in a surgical facility as an out-patient procedure without an overnight hospital stay. Anesthesia is used to numb the foot and ankle area and keep the patient awake but sedated. This anesthesia has longer lasting pain relief post-operatively and is less risky than spinal or general anesthesia. After surgery, the patient is given external supports like crutches or a walker with instructions to limit weight bearing on the affected foot. These supports are used from three to six weeks after surgery.

A compression dressing (Ace bandage) and a protective stiff-soled, Velcro strap-on shoe (Darco or cast shoe) are used. These are not very stylish post-op shoes, but they definitely are your friends. Occasionally, a cast is used for approximately six weeks where more protection is required. Modified shoe wear like sandals, cut out shoes, or extra depth shoes are usually wearable after six to eight weeks.

The average healing time for surgery when bones have been cut is usually eight weeks, although bone strengthening continues for the next year. You can expect to resume your sports and normal activities four to six months after surgery. Keep in mind that the foot is farthest from the heart. As a result, swelling is common. The most swelling occurs the first week, and it helps to elevate your foot higher than your heart. *Rest, ice,* and *elevation* are very important in the healing process, particularly during the acute phase. Do yourself a favor and follow those three simple treatments.

Swelling may persist for three to six months after surgery, and you may have to put off wearing your favorite gorgeous shoes for that long. Remember, bunion surgery is not a substitute for wearing shoes that fit!

Gale, a single thirty-year-old secretary, had bunion surgery six weeks earlier. Her stitches and surgical pin had been removed, and she arrived for her routine post-op appointment. Upon examination and x-ray, I found her great toe properly aligned and healing was taking place. She was quite unhappy and annoyed at me, however, because she had tried to wear her favorite dress pumps and her foot was still too swollen. She admitted that she had been informed that swelling was common for some time after foot surgery, but thought she would "snap back" right away.

She was pleased that her surgical result was good and was comforted that all was going well. I learned to provide written side effect information to the patient and to stress how common swelling is for several months after surgery. After another eight weeks, Gale could wear her favorite shoes for special occasions and agreed to lower heels and wider shoes for general wear. She has some mild stiffness in her toe but has regained full function.

Surgical Complications

No one wants to think about complications, but they do exist. Some of the common ones are:

- Fifteen to twenty percent of bunions recur some time after surgery.
- One to two percent risk of infection requires antibiotics and occasionally surgical draining.
- Stiffness may persist in the big toe even though the toe is better aligned than before surgery.
- Numbness around the big toe may occur, but is usually more of an annoyance than a real problem.
- The cut bone may not heal and could require a second procedure. This is unusual but can happen.

BUNIONETTES

Small toe bunions which have a high relationship to flat feet and tight heel cords are called bunionettes. A bunionette (or Tailor's bunion) commonly occurs in combination with big toe bunions. It does not progress in the same way as big toe bunions and is more easily treated by wearing properly fitting shoes. Shoes with extra depth (space), wide toe box and soft leather uppers, doughnut pads, and shoe stretching over the painful area are helpful. Bunionettes can be troublesome, causing secondary problems such as creating pressure and pain between the toes and ingrown nails.

Most bunionettes occur in women. The deformity and pressure from the bony bump that forms on the little toe can cause a painful callus on the outside of the foot. There may be pain under the toe and sole of the foot as well. The little toe may curl up and form a hammertoe. When this occurs, a painful callus develops on the top of this toe. Because the small toe is pushing or leaning against the fourth toe, soft or hard painful corns may develop between these toes.

Self-Help, Medical, and Surgical Treatment

The treatment of bunionettes is identical to those for big toe bunions. The surgical expectations and complications are also similar. Toe spacers of tube foam or lamb's wool, metatarsal pads, proper shoes, and arch supports are often of great help in relieving pain and pressure.

FIGURE 5-3. *Bunionette*

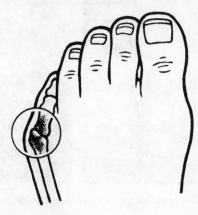

MALLET TOES, HAMMERTOES, AND CLAW TOES

If the tip of your toe (distal joint) is bent down towards the floor, the chances are you have a mallet toe. With mallet toes, a bump or corn forms on the top of this poor distal toe joint or a painful callus may appear at the tip of the same toe. In contrast to the mallet toe is the hammertoe (a hammertoe is not caused by dropping heavy objects like a hammer on the front part of the foot).

A hammertoe is an unusually contracted toe, bent at the middle portion of the toe (proximal interphalangeal joint, called the pip joint), and a bump and corn also appear on top of this toe. This usually develops over a period of years. It eventually reaches a point where it becomes obvious and painful. Most people do not notice its development until the area begins to hurt.

A claw toe is a combination of hammertoe and mallet toe with the extra added deformity at the base of the toe (the metatarsal phalangeal, MTP) joint. This is the joint as the base of toe close to the web space. The deformities shown in figure 5-4 are worth 1,000 words of description. The cause of most hammer or claw toes is unknown, but some are caused by systemic diseases or traumatic injuries. People with this condition have trouble finding comfortable shoes.

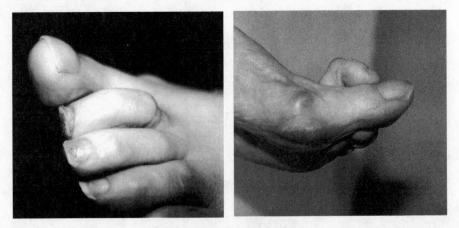

FIGURE 5-4. *Hammertoe, mallet toe (left), claw toe (right)*

Natural History

Why do these toes become deformed? Mallet toes, hammertoes, and claw toes can develop in isolated toes or multiple toes on one or both feet. They occur mostly in women and are most commonly found on the second toe (the toe next to the big toe), which is often longer than the other toes. The African tribal population of women who are usually shoeless demonstrate few incidents of these toe problems. There is a definite relationship between toe deformities and wearing improperly fitting shoes. Tight, too narrow, or too short shoes cause a buckling of the toe. They place constant abnormal pressure on the toes which makes them contract or twist. Women who wear shoes with four-inch spike heels and pointed toe boxes are probably headed for multiple deformities and problems.

There may also be a muscle imbalance between tendons on the top (extensor tendons) and bottom (flexor tendons) of the foot, causing toe deformities by pulling up or pulling down too much. Certain diseases like diabetes, Charcot Marie Tooth neuropathy, multiple sclerosis, herniated discs, or sciatica can also cause claw toes or hammertoes. Occasionally, when an injury happens to small muscles in the leg or foot, the scarring that results can cause toe deformities. There are some people who develop these problems from no known cause. Finally, bunions on the big toe may cause an overlap or underlap of the neighboring toes, and mallet toes, hammer toes, or claw toes will gradually form.

When you *first* notice a toe deformity like this on your feet, your toes are still flexible. They can still be moved into a straight position. You can see the deformity when you take a step and watch your toe curl up. Over time, the deformity will make the toe stiff and inflexible. At this point, you will see that you cannot straighten it out. So self examination and early detection are extremely important. If unsure, contact your doctor.

Symptoms

Mallet toe pain comes from the callus that forms on the tip of the toe as a result of its bending downward and rubbing against the shoe. Nail problems also develop from hitting the shoe. If you have a hammertoe, you will most likely find upon examination a large callus on the top of this toe. It usually causes pain when it hits the shoe. See chapter 6 for a detailed discussion of calluses and corns.

The claw toe sufferer will experience the same toe pain and a callus will also form on the metatarsal pad of the foot under the metatarsal head. The Metatarsophalangeal (MTP) joint can become inflamed and occasionally unstable. Instability can cause the MTP joint to dislocate, swell (top and bottom of ball of foot), and become very painful. This claw toe condition is common in people with rheumatoid arthritis, diabetes, or other nerve problems, or when foot and leg muscles have been injured causing contractures and muscle imbalances.

Self-Help Treatment

Mallet toe deformities can sometimes be helped with the use of a toe crest placed under the middle of the toe. This lifts the toe up and relieves pressure from the toe tip. Hammertoes cause pain at the top of the toe. A hammertoe strap pulls this toe down more in line. Tube foam or mole-

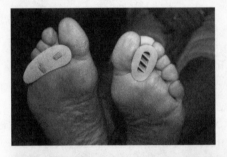

skin placed over the toe will help cushion it from hitting the shoe. Most important, the shoes you wear must be wide and deep enough to fit your toe deformity. High heels and pointed shoes aggravate the toes by bending them and increasing pressure.

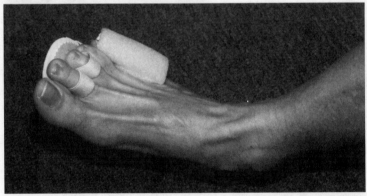

FIGURE 5-5A. *Toe spacer on right foot (bunion) and toe crest on left foot (mallet toe)*

FIGURE 5-5B. *Hammer toe strap and tube foam (protective padding)*

Metatarsal pads placed in the shoe behind the metatarsal pad on the foot will lift the metatarsal heads some and may alleviate pain by helping straighten the toes. See figure 5-5.

Medical Treatment

A medical evaluation is essential if toe deformities are caused by diseases. A neurologist will often be the best choice depending on the disease. NSAIDs can reduce swelling and pain. A shoe prescription like a stiff sole rocker shoe helps relieve pressure at the MTP joint by rocking the foot over the joint during walking. This changes your gait and the toe joints are not bent as much. See chapter 15 on shoes.

Surgical Treatment

When should you have an operation to correct your toe deformity? The best answer is when shoes and various straps, pads, and so on, do not relieve your pain and reasonable shoes are uncomfortable. At this point it is probably time to surgically correct and straighten your toes.

Surgery combines soft tissue release or loosening of joint ligaments and transferring tendons to rebalance the muscle pulling power in the toes. There are no associated problems with the alteration of these tendons. Shortening the toe by removing some bone at the joint may be necessary as well. Hammer and mallet toes require a straightening and stiffening at the Proximal Interphalangeal joint (PIP) or distal joint. A small surgical pin is usually placed in the toe and extends out of the tip. This allows the toe to stiffen in a straight position. A ball is placed on the end of the pin. The pin is easily (and usually painlessly) removed in the office three to six weeks after surgery.

In a claw toe, the PIP joint is straightened in the same way. In addition, the Metatarsophalangeal (MTP) joint's tight ligaments need to be released. This procedure eliminates clawing at the joint. Sometimes, tendons are transferred for balance as well.

Remember, if a bunion on the big toe is contributing to these other toe deformities, it is necessary to surgically correct this problem because it is part of the deforming cause. In general, surgical expectations are the same as after post-op bunion surgery.

Helen, a 65-year-old retired teacher, came to see me with complaints of disabling pain over the top of her second toe. She was even having trouble wearing her wide walking shoes. She explained that her mother had experienced foot problems, as well.

Examination and x-rays showed a severely angled, great toe bunion deformity on her right foot. While standing, the great toe was underlying the second toe pushing it upward. A painfully inflamed callus was present on the top of her second toe and another callus was on the tip of this toe. The hammertoe was caused by her great toe bunion. She had tried shoe modifications and straps without success.

Since the symptoms were very painful and progressive in nature, she elected to have surgical correction to straighten the great toe and second toe. She had a good result without complications and her calluses disappeared three months after the pressure was relieved. She can walk comfortably in her sport shoes and continues to do well.

Swelling can be a problem as it limits shoe wear. Less time is spent on crutches than with bunion surgery and casts are rarely used. A stiff sole shoe and dressings are worn. The sutures are usually removed at two weeks and the surgical pins are removed in the doctor's office after three to six weeks. Rest, elevation, and ice are always helpful to healing.

IN A NUTSHELL

A bunion is a big toe that is misaligned at the joint. Bunions often have no symptoms and most bunion pain is caused by faulty fitting shoewear. When bunions progress and worsen, they may develop painful symptoms and can cause secondary problems like hammertoes on other toes. Bunionettes are bunions of the small toe and if symptomatic are treated like bunions. Shoe devices and proper shoes should be tried first before surgery is considered.

Hammertoes, mallet toes, and claw toes can exist on their own or as the result of a great toe bunion. There are many shoe devices and shoe modifications that can help take pressure off these toes. Surgery to correct these deformities can be performed if they worsen and other measures don't help. This surgery is quite successful.

DOCTOR'S CORNER: QUESTIONS AND ANSWERS

Should I have bunion surgery right away? My doctor advised me to have my bunion operated on during my first visit.

Foot surgery is almost always elective. It means you have time on your side to try other ways to improve your symptoms like wider, extra depth shoes, toe spacers, arch supports, metatarsal pads, and orthotics. When your bunion cannot be accommodated by any of these methods and the pain continues or the bunion deformity gets worse, you should consider surgical correction. *It is important for you to feel comfortable with and have confidence in your doctor.*

Several of my friends have told me not to have bunion surgery because it doesn't work. My bunions are preventing me from getting around and enjoying life. So, what should I do?

Surgical techniques and training in bunion surgery have improved dramatically in the past few years. It is also important to remember that bunion surgery helps correct secondary symptoms like hammertoes, mallet toes, or claw toes by removing abnormal pressures against these other toes. Also, bunions often make your symptoms worse. Bunion surgery is usually done under a local anesthetic, and significant complications are rare. Don't forget that you still will need to wear shoes that give enough room to your feet, even after bunion surgery.

I've got a bunion, two hammertoes, and a corn on my small toe—all on the same foot. The bunion hurts but the other toes don't. My husband says I should have all these corrected at the same time. What should I do?

In general, foot surgery is done for progressive and/or painful deformities after other self-help care and medical treatments have been tried and failed. It is usually better to operate on just the toe which has symptoms. It is understood that the more surgery you have, the greater the chance for complications. An example of an exception to this would be a non-symptomatic bunion that causes PAINFUL symptoms in other toes. Correcting your painful bunion will relieve the pressures on the other toes, as well.

TERMS TO REMEMBER

Arthrodesis (fusion): The elimination of a specific joint or foot motion by locking bones together to gain stabilization and to eliminate pain.

Bunion: A bump, abnormality, or a deviation of the big toe joint that is misaligned and caused by abnormal pressure.

Bunionette: A small toe bunion.

Claw toe: A combination of hammertoe and mallet toe, caused by abnormal pressures or buckling at both toe joints.

Distal joints: Joints in the toe closest to the nail.

Extensor tendons: Tendons on the top of the foot that lift (extend) the toes off the floor.

Flexor tendons: Tendons that are attached to muscles that curl the toes toward the floor.

Hammertoe: A deformed toe that buckles up at the middle toe joint.

Keller procedure: A specific bunion or great toe arthritis operation that removes half of the joint to relieve pressure and/or realign the joint. It is not used as commonly now as in the past.

Lateral: The outside of the foot or leg; the "little toe" side.

Mallet toe: A deformed toe that is bent under at the end toe joint.

Medial: The midline or inside of the foot or leg; the "big toe" side of the foot.

Modified McBride procedure: A soft tissue surgical ligament release and tightening procedure to correct a bunion.

NSAID: Non-steroidal anti-inflammatory medicine is a general term for medicines that treat inflammation, pain, and swelling. Most are prescription medicines, but some are over-the-counter. All can cause side effects, primarily involving the stomach or intestine.

Phalanx: Singular of phalanges; one of the small bones of the toes.

Proximal interphalangeal (PIP) joint: The joints in the middle of the toes.

CHAPTER 6

Metatarsalgia, Calluses, Corns, and Warts

INTRODUCTION

A typical scenario I hear in my office from patients with problems of this sort is, *"The ball of my foot hurts, Doctor, and I have a thick callus there, too. I also have a small, very painful corn on the tip of my toe where it curls down."* Since so many of these symptoms are interconnected with the problems of metatarsalgia, calluses, corns, and warts, these problems are grouped together. Warts, a virus infection, are often misdiagnosed as calluses and are included for that reason.

Among the more painful adult foot problems are metatarsalgia, calluses, corns, and warts. If you have such problems, they should be diagnosed and promptly treated. Evaluate your shoes in line with your occupation. Get medical help as needed.

WHAT IS METATARSALGIA?

Metatarsalgia, like fluid on the knee, is not a diagnosis but a symptom of another problem. It is a painful condition located across or localized to the ball of the foot (metatarsal pad). It feels like there is a stone in your shoe. *Algia* means pain and quite frequently is directly related to the basic structure of the foot. For example, a high arch (cavus) foot, claw toes, and a tightness or deformity in the ankle or hindfoot which transmits pressure to the heel (tight heel cords) are frequently associated. See figure 6-1.

Metatarsalgia can also be caused by frequent wearing of high heel shoes. Occasionally, it is part of a systemic illness or injury such as rheumatoid arthritis, diabetes, certain muscle diseases, or traumatic injuries which result in deformed bones. In these cases, the initial problem begins with the loss of nerve and/or muscle function leading to imbalance or inflammation of the ball joint (metatarsal phalangeal joint). These deformities may still be flexible, but eventually the joints become

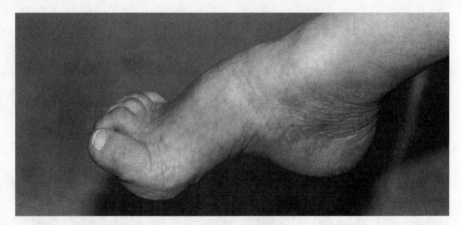

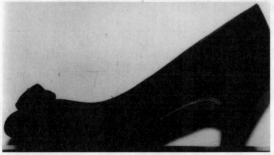

FIGURE 6-1. *High arch (pes cavus) and high heel*

fixed and stiff. The arch ligament becomes tight and one or more of the metatarsal bones point downward. The ball of the foot becomes callused and the toes claw (curl up). The normal padding in the ball of the foot wears thin and the foot can no longer tolerate the normal amount of stress. You may blame the calluses as the problem, but in fact they are the tip of the iceberg. See figure 6-2.

THE MENACING CALLUS, CORN, AND WART

Calluses

Our skin loses its elasticity as we grow older, making it susceptible to corns, calluses, ulcers, and infection. These problems are often aggravated by ill-fitting shoes or functional imbalance in one's foot or leg. A callus (or corn) is a thickening of the skin caused by recurring friction or pressure on the skin caught between bone and an adjacent firm surface like a shoe, the floor, and so on. The skin is attempting to adapt to this abnormal pressure by becoming thicker.

Unfortunately, as the protective response continues, the formed callus becomes thicker and less flexible. It takes up even more space in your

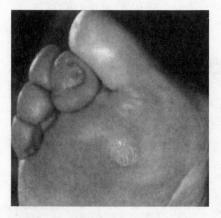

shoe and eventually will become inflamed. Usually, this thickened skin is not painful, unless pressure is directly applied to it. Just by walking or standing, the ball of the foot has pressure applied to it about 60 percent of the time. This is the prime area where most calluses form. You will notice them when they are thicker and less flexible because they become more painful.

FIGURE 6-2. *Severe bunion and callus; great toe rotated 70° with associated multiple toe deformities*

Calluses are common in people who walk barefoot and also among those who stand on their feet all day, especially on rough hard surfaces. They are usually the sign of structural or incorrect weight distribution. For example, women who wear high-heel shoes tend to push body weight on the ball of the foot, causing calluses in the area.

Corns

A corn, like a callus, is a thickening of the skin which is a response to pressure. Corns are usually found on the sides of the feet, between the toes, or on top of a hammer or mallet toe. Repeated friction aggravates the toe or the irritated area and accelerates the cell production of cornified skin. The corn actually develops to protect the irritated area. But,

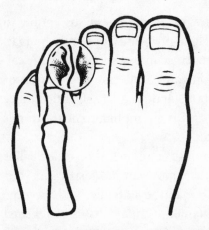

unfortunately, the deeper the corn grows the more likely it is to irritate a nerve that transmits the pain you feel. A common location for a corn is between the toes, usually the fourth and fifth toe. It appears as either a

FIGURE 6-3. *Corn between toes (left),* *Corns from hammer and mallet toes (below)*

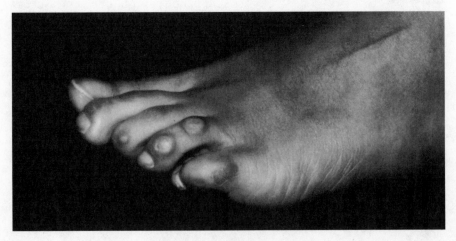

firm, thickening skin, or it can be soft. Occasionally, it ulcerates, a result of the side pressure of one toe pressing against another. See figure 6-3.

Warts

A wart, often mistaken for a callus, is a skin growth caused by a virus found on the bottom of the foot. Minor cuts or fissures in the foot are perfect entry points for the virus. A wart appears as an area of thickened, elevated, irregular skin. It frequently has small dark markings within the center. These marks are small blood vessels which will bleed when the wart is scraped. The diagnosis of a wart is made by observing these vessels. The

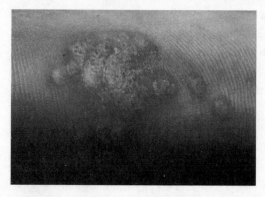

wart may or may not be painful. Sometimes the pain may be caused by squeezing it from side to side instead of from direct pressure. Even without treatment, they frequently clear up in a few months. See figure 6-4.

FIGURE 6-4. *Mosaic wart*

E velyn, an active seventy-five-year-old woman living in a retirement community, came to my office because of a growth between the fourth and fifth toes on her left foot. It had disrupted her life because of the disabling pain it caused. The area sometimes drained, and she was worried about infection.

The examination showed thickened corns on the inside of both her toes. They were pressing against each other and there were bony prominences under each corn. She had tried lambswool and corn pads and had adjusted her shoe size and style. None of these measures helped her symptoms.

She elected surgery. Under local anesthetic, the small bony prominences were removed, which relieved the pressure causing her corns. After healing, Evelyn was able to resume her community dancing and other activities, wearing comfortable shoes.

J eff, a twenty-year-old college intramural athlete, arrived at my clinic complaining of a painful wart on his foot that wouldn't go away. He had been treated by another physician who had done intermittent shaving and treating of the wart with salicylic acid for a period of four months. He got only temporary relief and the thickened tissue recurred within about three weeks. The wart was only painful when he walked on it.

Upon examination, I found a thickened whitish elevated tissue on the bottom of his plantar pad. When I applied direct pressure to the area, it caused pain but squeezing it wasn't painful. An anatomical examination of his foot revealed a prominent etatarsal bone that pushed into this thickened skin area. X-rays showed an old fracture that had healed in a slightly bent position and caused abnormal pressure on the area producing a callus.

This problem was not a wart at all, but a callus. Metatarsal pads were tried to relieve pressure, but the symptoms worsened. Jeff elected to have an osteotomy (a controlled breaking) of the metatarsal bone to correct the malalignment and relieve pressure. His callus cleared up when healing took place and no further treatment was necessary. Jeff experienced no more pain symptoms and resumed his sports program.

Note: *Warts often appear on nonbony prominences of the foot. They have brownish spots which are small capillaries that carry the blood supply for the wart. Calluses don't have these spots and usually are painful when pressure is applied.*

Symptoms

Calluses are caused by the pressure of an underlying bone and are not painful at rest. They are painful when they begin to put pressure on the nerve or blood supply beneath it. Narrow or high-heel narrow toe shoes will aggravate the callus. The pressure is actually from the foot bones contacting the floor during walking. When calluses appear on both feet and across the whole metatarsal pad, there is usually a problem in the heel or ankle, or they have been triggered by another medical problem.

A single large callus usually means the presence of a long metatarsal bone or some other anatomical variant. A seed-like small callus or corn suggests a larger metatarsal head than normal, causing localized pressure. Diffuse swelling of the metatarsal pad requires comparing both feet. When swelling is present but no large callus exists, the condition suggests joint inflammation either from localized overstress or a medical problem such as rheumatoid arthritis. The pad or ball of the foot will be swollen, as will, in many cases, the top of the foot at the base of the toes. This disease begins as a joint lining swelling and inflammation.

The pain from metatarsalgia, or joint swelling, must also be differentiated from a Morton's neuroma. There is tenderness from a neuroma when you push on the painful area and the pain is between the metatarsal bones, not directly beneath the bone. Tingling or numbness is frequently present when a neuroma is the problem.

Secondary symptoms to look for when you have a painful callus somewhere else on the foot include:

- High arch (tight arch ligaments) leading to arch inflammation (plantar fasciatis).

- Tight heel cords with pain localized to the heel cord (Achilles tendon) and aggravated by jumping or standing on your toes.

- Deformed, stiff ankle or hindfoot from arthritis or injury.

- Hip or knee arthritis with limited motion which puts abnormal stress on the foot.

Self-Help Treatment

Mild corns can be treated without medical remedies. The simplest approach, of course, is to look for the cause and eliminate it. If changing shoes does not help, then place pads with a hole to clear the corn, preventing friction between the corn and the shoe. Once the pressure on the corn or callus is eliminated, the callus will disappear over a few weeks to several months.

There are a myriad of over-the-counter remedies which should be evaluated with caution. Mostly, all corn remedies are caustic and cause severe burns or blisters.

Before looking into a quick remedy, make sure that pressure on a callus triggers the pain. Here are some self-help hints that you should consider:

- Reevaluate your foot size, shape, and stiffness, and make the necessary adjustments in your shoe wear. The key words are extra depth, wider toe box, and lower heels.

- Metatarsal pads in the proper place in the shoe to lift the painful area or soft insole inserts like Spenko or Dr. Scholl's may decrease but not eliminate pressure symptoms.

- Wearing soft-soled shoes and creating a soft-standing surface (rubber mats in the work space) may relieve callus, knee, or back pain.

- Try arch supports purchased over the counter, and see how well they relieve the pressure or pain.

Lillian, a middle-aged salesperson, saw me at my clinic with a complaint of pain from thickened calluses across the ball of her foot. She experienced pain when she walked and when she wore her high heels at work.

At her examination, I found abnormally high arches on both feet and she had calluses under all the metatarsal heads across the ball of her feet. She had tight arch ligaments (plantar fascia) and metatarsalgia caused from her high arch anatomy.

This caused her metatarsal bones to angle down to the floor, creating pain and abnormal pressure. I fitted her with soft arch supports to cushion her foot providing shock absorption. I also put metatarsal pads behind the calluses to change pressure away from her metatarsal bones. She was encouraged to wear lower heel, extra depth, wider toe shoes.

These treatments provided her with relief from pain, and she only felt discomfort when she had to wear formal shoes for special occasions.

Since the size of the callus may cause pain, you can control the overgrowth of this thick tissue by soaking the affected area in warm water and then filing down the callus with a pumice stone for one to two minutes as needed. You can also use a callus razor, making sure you trim the callus only to the level of the adjacent skin. Cutting too deeply carries the danger of a disastrous infection and is generally not recommended. Diabetic patients and people with limited mobility, decreased eyesight, or limited dexterity should NOT trim their own calluses.

The best self-help for warts is to prevent them from occurring. Small cuts on the feet puncture the skin and serve as an entry point for the virus. Use proper shoe protection. Do not walk barefoot in risky environments. Properly clean and cover small cuts. Most warts disappear in four or five months without any treatment. Painful, large, or multiple warts should be medically treated.

How to Locate the Metatarsal Pad in Your Shoe

Here is one procedure to follow in locating the metatarsal pad in your shoe:

- Carefully feel the bottom of your foot to find the areas of maximum tenderness. These are usually found directly under a hard bone in the ball of your foot.

- Mark the tender areas with a marker such as lipstick or a color that clearly contrasts with that of the shoe insoles. See figure 6-5.

- Place your bare foot inside the shoe and take a few steps to leave marks.

- Remove the shoe and locate the marks.

- Remove the paper from the sticky surface of the Hapad, a cushioned metatarsal pad that is semifirm in design. Its purpose is to take pressure off the metatarsal head. Situate the hapad in the shoe so that the edge of the hapad almost butts against the side of the spots on the bottom of the shoe.

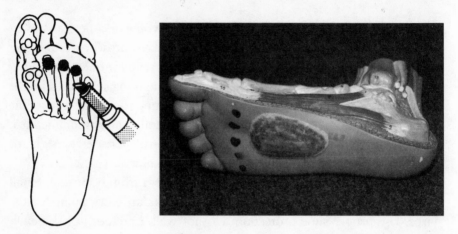

FIGURE 6-5. *Locating metatarsal pads and pad placement (normally on shoe or arch support)*

Medical Treatment

Problem calluses may be the result of conditions elsewhere in the limbs like stiff hips, arthritis or other knee problems, and tight heel cords. The back, hips, knees, ankles, and feet need to be examined and appropriate x-rays should be taken. A physician familiar with the mechanical working of the whole leg should be contacted.

Pressure-relieving devices like custom-molded orthotics, shoe sole alterations, wedges or metatarsal bars, a rocker sole, or stiff shank may be prescribed. Occasionally, patients are required to wear customized shoes for severe deformities. This is especially true for those with rheumatic or diabetic foot problems, since they are severe and take multiple forms. Fortunately, the shoe industry has come up with a variety of footware that accommodates most foot problems at less cost than custom shoes. See chapter 15 on the proper shoes to wear. Consult a pedorthist (specialist in shoe fitting and accommodations) when fitting is a problem.

Custom-molded orthotics are commonly prescribed, but proper shoes must accommodate these orthotics. If the callus is related to a high arch, stiff tight foot, a soft device is prescribed. Occasionally, a rigid or plastic support is recommended if the callus problem is secondary to abnormal motion. These devices are expensive and cannot be guaranteed to solve the problem. Consider this carefully before you invest in them. Trimming a callus when skin growth is excessive usually helps.

Your doctor may also try a variety of the pressure-relieving devices described in the self-help section.

Wart treatment depends on the diagnosis. A cursory look at the small central core with its blood vessels identifies it as a wart. But such a core is sometimes overgrown by thick skin and cannot be diagnosed correctly. Trimming the outer skin creates bleeding which can determine that a wart exists. In contrast, trimming a callus does not cause bleeding.

Most warts disappear in a few months and two-thirds are gone within two years. Therefore, it is important not to overtreat warts. For isolated or multiple small warts, a forty percent salicylic acid plaster or a fifty percent trichlorocilic acid should do the job. Other chemical agents may be prescribed in difficult cases. In any case, you must protect the surrounding skin by using a moleskin doughnut cut out with only the wart exposed to the medication. A second moleskin section can cover the wart for protection after treatment. The patient can apply the treatment each evening, soak the foot the following morning, and gently rub the wart with a pumice stone, emory board, or stiff washcloth. Treatment should continue until the skin is smooth and no tiny pin-prick dots of blood vessels are visible.

Surgical Treatment

When painful calluses do not respond to other treatment, then the patient is a candidate for surgical treatment. The first step is to identify the cause of the abnormal pressure. It could be that the callus under the second toe is caused by stress transferred from the large bunion on the great toe. Correcting the bunion problem will redistribute the pressure and cause the callus to disappear.

A long and isolated callus under the second toe suggests that the second metatarsal bone is long. If symptoms cannot be controlled medically, this bone may have to be shortened. Unfortunately, when one metatarsal bone is shortened or its angulation changed by an osteotomy, there is the chance of a transfer callus to another toe. Therefore, symptoms must be severe enough and self-help and medical treatment exhausted before this somewhat unpredictable procedure is performed.

If the metatarsal pain is related to a claw toe, it can often be relieved by straightening the hammertoe and releasing the tight tendons and ligaments. Pain located between the metatarsal (second and third or third and fourth toes) is often caused by Morton's neuroma, see chapter 7. Removal of this swollen nerve should relieve the symptoms. The small fifth toe sometimes will have a callus under the metatarsal pad caused by a bunionette. Correcting this deformity by cutting and reangulating the bone will cure this callus problem.

One cannot always blame all pain under the metatarsal head on the bone pressure. Pain may be secondary to an inflamed MTP (metatarsal phalangeal) joint or a dislocated joint. Subtle swelling (not a callus) may be noticed in this area. Flexing and extending the toe up and down will cause pain as well. This is in contrast to callus pain caused by direct pressure rather than toe motion. Surgery to remove the inflamed joint lining (**synovectomy**) along with tightening the joint ligaments (possibly rerouting some tendons) may be required.

When calluses are located across the entire forefoot, isolated bone surgeries would only result in transferring pain to another area. Medical treatment should be adequate, although a procedure to correct the structure of the foot is considered. For example, cutting the heel bone (os calcis) to change its angulation alters pressure on the toes. Cutting the tight arch ligament (plantar fascia) will also decrease the pulling pressure on the metatarsal bones. When hips or knees have an abnormal alignment from arthritis or injury, total hip or total knee replacements may relieve foot stresses.

Inasmuch as most warts can be treated with self-help and drugs, some warts may require surgical treatment. Liquid nitrogen (cryosurgery or freezing) is the most common wart surgery. Surgical curettage to pare the wart down is sometimes used. Laser excision is becoming more popular, as well. It has been known to accurately remove the wart tissue without damage to adjacent tissue. Surgical excision, however, is rarely used on warts located on the weight bearing (sole) part of the foot. There is more risk of scarring with this procedure. Scars of the bottom of the foot are notoriously painful and difficult to treat.

All these procedures have a 25-40 percent chance of recurrence of the wart or less than complete elimination of the original wart. Further surgery or alternate treatments often follow.

IN A NUTSHELL

Metatarsalgia is a painful condition on the ball of the foot. Often, calluses are found in this area, as well. If you have a corn or a callus, you should know that they are thickened skin that develops as a reaction to abnormal pressures from things like bony prominences, faulty fitting shoes, high arches, and so on. The causes of the corns and calluses need to be diagnosed and treated by your doctor.

Warts are often mistaken for calluses. They are caused by a virus and usually have tiny blood vessel marks on them. A variety of treatments are used for warts, but they will sometimes clear up on their own over time.

DOCTOR'S CORNER: QUESTIONS AND ANSWERS

I need to trim my corns every few weeks when they start to hurt. Should I do anything else to them?

You need to be very careful trimming your corns so that you don't cause infection. If you are a diabetic or have vascular disease, DON'T trim your own corns. Get professional help for this problem. The cause of your corns needs to be determined, since often simple shoe alterations and/or shoe inserts will relieve pressure. The corns will often be diminished in size, become less painful, or disappear altogether, as a result.

I have several painful calluses on the ball of my foot. What kind of surgery would fix this problem?

I assume that you have already tried appropriate shoe alterations and inserts without success before surgery was considered. You need to have the mechanics of your entire foot evaluated. If only one or two metatarsal bones are angled too much into the metatarsal pad, cutting these bones to relieve pressure may be done (osteotomies). However, with this procedure the stress can be transferred to other metatarsals and isn't as successful as other surgeries.

If calluses are across the ball of your foot, you may have high arches which suggest mechanical problems that involve more of your foot. This could include a tight arch ligament, tight heel cords, and an abnormally angled heel bone. Cutting the plantar ligament to relieve tension, cutting the heel bone to change its angle, and changing the metatarsal bone angles may be necessary for a successful outcome. It is a complex problem with many surgical alternatives.

TERMS TO REMEMBER

Callus: A thickening of the skin caused by recurring friction or pressure on the skin caught between bone and an adjacent firm surface like a shoe or the floor.

Cavus: A foot with a high arch.

Corn: A callus usually found on the side of the feet, between the toes, or on top of a hammer or mallet toe.

Hapad: A cushioned metatarsal pad. Its purpose is to take pressure off the metatarsal head.

Metatarsalgia: A painful condition, usually on the ball of the foot.

Synovectomy: Surgery to remove an inflamed joint lining that often includes the rerouting of tendons.

Wart: A skin growth caused by a virus found on the bottom of the foot; an area of thickened, elevated, irregular skin.

CHAPTER 7

What Should I Do About My Morton's Neuroma?

INTRODUCTION

Nerves are conductors of sensation, stimulate muscle function, control the perspiration and skin temperature, and assist in regulating circulation. There are nerve problems that occur in the foot and ankle which can cause serious and painful conditions. The first such problem is a neuroma. Strictly speaking, a neuroma is a tumor. But when we speak of a neuroma of a nerve, we refer to inflammation of the nerve or the tissue surrounding the nerve. An irritated nerve is caused by abnormal pressure

Dealing with nerve problems is not an easy job. The last thing you want is surgery. Morton's neuroma and tarsal tunnel can be treated by proper shoes and metatarsal pads. If you suspect Reflex Sympathetic Dystrophy (RSD), early medical treatment is very important to avoid prolonged complications.

from bones, surrounding tissue, traumatic injuries, or surgical injuries. When nerves are partially or totally cut, they try to regenerate. This attempt usually fails. The newly formed nerve tissue swells and heads in the wrong direction. Scar tissue forms around it and causes added pressure on the new nerve tissue.

Any nerve in the foot can be injured and form a neuroma. But the most common foot nerve problems is Morton's neuroma which we will discuss later in the chapter. The nerves of the foot are illustrated in figure 7-1.

NERVE PROBLEMS

A neuroma can occur anywhere there is a nerve in the body. The affected nerve is pinched or entrapped for a variety of reasons. For example, it is common for a tight or narrow toe box shoe to pinch a nerve. The most common neuroma in the foot is found between the third and fourth toes. A burning, tingling, or pins-and-needles sensation is frequently associated with nerve symptoms.

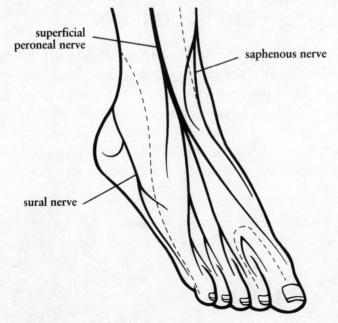

FIGURE 7-1. *Nerves of the foot*

Other nerve problems have many causes—often a result of nerve disease or injury elsewhere in the body. For example, a herniated disc in the back can cause referred pain that frequently radiates down to the foot. Tightness or scarring in the ligament tunnels, which nerves pass through, causes nerve pain to the foot. Tarsal tunnel (ligament behind the ankle) is the most common example of this condition in the foot. You are probably more familiar with a similar condition called carpal tunnel in the wrist. The tarsel tunnel compresses on the nerve, causing radiating pain in the foot (sometimes just to the big toe, sometimes to the bottom of the entire foot, or other variations). A signal of a nerve problem is a tingling sensation when you tap on the irritated nerve. This is called a tinel sign. The tingling radiates away from the irritated area of the nerve into the foot or up into the leg.

A third nerve condition in the foot and leg is RSD (reflex sympathetic dystrophy) or causalgia (pain) syndrome. Unlike other nerve conditions which affect muscle or sensory function (feeling pin prick, light touch), RSD affects the autonomic nervous system which involves our sympathetic and para-sympathetic nerves. These small nerves travel with other nerves but are not under our voluntary control. They primarily control the amount of circulation to the feet and shivering or sweating response. They also keep our skin moist and lubricated.

There are medical conditions that cause nerve problems to the foot. These include thyroid disease, arthritis conditions, rheumatoid arthritis, lupus, or peripheral vascular disease. These conditions may cause swelling and could lead to tunnel compression and nerve pain. Diabetes can also affect the nerves of the foot through many symptoms, including loss of sensation. See chapter 10 which elaborates on the diabetic foot.

MORTON'S NEUROMA

The key question often asked is "How do I know I have Morton's neuroma? Morton's neuroma (also called interdigital neuroma) is seven times more common in women than men. It appears more frequently when tight shoes or high heels are worn regularly. It also can appear after foot injuries occur, or for no apparent reason at all. Often these patients recall a preexisting injury to the big toe. It shows up mostly in middle age and there is an increased incidence in runners and dancers. An athlete with hypermobile (loose ligaments) foot and excessive pronation is a candidate for this disorder.

At first, Morton's neuroma symptoms occur in weight bearing, but eventually happen even at rest. Removing the shoes or lowering the height of the heel will help take the weight off the nerve area. See figure 7-2.

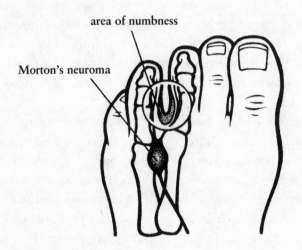

FIGURE 7-2. *Morton's neuroma*

Key Symptoms

The most common symptoms of Morton's neuroma are:

- Pain on the bottom of the foot under the pad of the third or fourth toe, or occasionally between the second and third toes. There is also burning pain into the third and fourth toes. Pain is increased by walking and is relieved by removing the shoes or by resting.

- Burning or sharp, cramping pain.

- Numbness and tingling in the foot or toes.

- Pain that radiates to one or two toes.

- Inflammation with associated swelling.

Self-Help Treatment

To benefit from quick and simple relief, we recommend the following measures:

- Wear extra depth and low heel shoes to relieve pressure on the nerves.
- Cushion type of insoles like Spenko brand may help.
- Discontinue running or other activities that might have set off this problem.
- Wear small metatarsal pads behind the involved area to assist in spreading bones of the foot apart.
- Use orthotics incorporating the metatarsal pads.

Medical Treatment

If these measures do not help, then you need a medical doctor to review your shoe wear. He or she may give you a local injection of cortisone and anesthetic for quick relief. It will help a lot to let your doctor know the effect of the treatment. Injections are not repeated that often and frequently are only of temporary benefit. They are helpful, however, in confirming the diagnosis. If pain is temporarily relieved by accurately placing the Xylocaine (Novocaine) over the nerve, it is confirmation that a neuroma exists. An ultrasound exam or an MRI can also help diagnose the problem, but are rarely recommended.

Surgical Help

In terms of surgery, a Morton's neuroma surgical procedure typically removes the swollen nerve and releases the ligaments that have caused pressure and pain between the toes. You can expect dramatic relief. Wearing proper shoes is also critical for preventing recurrence.

Surgical Expectations

There is approximately an eighty percent chance of dramatic relief. As the soft tissues heal, crutches are used for two to three weeks. The patient begins to gain mobility during this time. Keep in mind the risk associated with nerve surgery. It is possible that pain will not be relieved and may worsen because new neuromas appear. With a second surgery, there is a seventy-five percent chance of success. Neuromas can show up in any area of the foot from cuts, including after surgery. The bone may need shaving to relieve pressure or to free the nerve from scar tissue. Healing is a bit slower in these cases and the success rate is not as predictable. On occasion, a new neuroma will form where the previous

Claire, a thirty-five-year-old conference planner, arrived at my office with severe pain on the bottom of the outside pad of her foot (plantar pad). She stated that after she had worn her work heels on a hard floor surface for a long work day, she experienced pain and numbness between the third and fourth toes on her right foot. It became even more painful when she tried to wear high heel shoes. She even experienced pain when she walked barefoot on the sand on a recent beach trip.

My examination of her foot showed no abnormal calluses on her plantar pad. I carefully probed her toes and she experienced pain between the metatarsal bones of her third and fourth toes. When I squeezed the ball of her foot together, she felt increased pain and a clicking sensation. I injected the area between her third and fourth toes with Xylocaine (a Novocaine derivative) and cortisone. She experienced immediate relief.

I diagnosed her problem as a Morton's neuroma. I also placed metatarsal pads in her shoes to relieve pressure and encouraged her to wear extra depth, low heeled shoes except for special occasions. After about three weeks, her pain symptoms recurred.

After another four months of disabling foot pain, she elected to have surgery to remove her painful swollen nerve. She experienced immediate relief and within about three weeks, was walking comfortably in her low heel shoes.

Note: *The most common location for Morton's neuroma is between the third and fourth toes. The next most common area is between the second and third toes. It is rarely located between other toes unless there has been a nerve injury to the area.*

nerve was cut. If this occurs, repeat conservative care, injections, or nerve medicine. Pads are again tried before surgery is repeated. Unfortunately, on occasion all nerve pain cannot be relieved, and you must live with and adjust to your symptoms.

TARSAL TUNNEL

The problem of tarsal tunnel in the foot is similar to the more common carpal tunnel problem in the wrist. They often occur together or one may develop later. The ligament around the inside of the ankle tightens and presses on the major nerve (posterior tibial nerve) to the foot. This is caused by a tightening of the ligament around the tunnel through which this nerve passes. People with flat feet experience it often, because their ankles roll out (pronate), putting tension on the inside of the ankle ligaments.

Tarsal tunnel can also occur in high arched feet with tight ligaments. Trauma to the foot (even minor injuries) and medical conditions which cause swelling may compress the tunnel as well. This is a tougher problem to diagnose than carpal tunnel, because the symptoms are often generalized aches in the foot. Pain is characterized by cramping and burning which is worse at night, as in carpal tunnel syndrome. An index of sus-

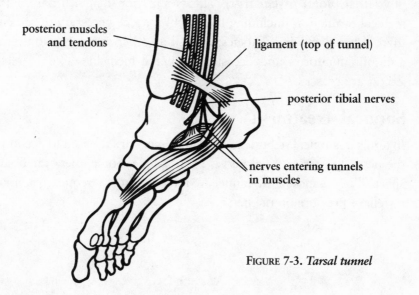

posterior muscles and tendons

ligament (top of tunnel)

posterior tibial nerves

nerves entering tunnels in muscles

FIGURE 7-3. *Tarsal tunnel*

picion (awareness, sensitivity, and knowledge of diseases that are elusive, hard to diagnose, or are often overlooked) must be employed in diagnosing tarsal tunnel.

Self-Help Treatment

The simplest self-help step is wearing comfortable shoes with adequate support to relieve pressure areas. Arch supports can also be used to lift and minimize pressure in some cases. Limiting activities, rest, ice, and elevation should provide welcome relief. Patients are advised to document the activities, shoes, etc. that make the problem worse and pay close attention to how the pain feels, where it radiates, and so forth. This much monitoring will make it easier for the doctor to home in on the problem and prescribe the right cure.

Medical Help

People with excessively pronated feet may have to wear custom orthotics by prescription. High arches may need a soft shock absorbing support. If the condition worsens, you should get a medical evaluation to determine the cause of your nerve problem. Nerve and muscle testing using EMG and nerve conduction testing are the specialty of a neurologist or physiatrist (*not* a psychiatrist). This is real, not imagined pain. Further medical evaluation (including lab work) may be necessary to search for thyroid problems and diabetes, as well as other ailments. Nonsteroidal anti-inflammatories and occasionally nerve medicines like Tegretal or Zoloft are prescribed.

Surgical Treatment

In terms of surgical treatment, the tight tissues are released to decompress the nerve (posterior tibial nerve) at the ankle. Sometimes scar tissue or space filling tissues in the tunnel are removed (most frequently a lipoma) to relieve pressure on the nerve.

Surgical Expectations

After surgery, a cast or splint is usually worn for about six weeks. Crutches are also used. Rest and elevation are important during recovery. You may expect numbness and tingling to persist due to inflammation and swelling from surgery. This condition may last for several months and can, on occasion, be permanent. If the corrected problem was tarsal tunnel, there is a seventy-five percent chance of relief from pain. It is hard to predict the success of this type of surgery, as it can be only partially relieved. The tarsal tunnel may be combined with back problems, other medical conditions, or foot mechanical problems like flat feet or high arches. If these conditions are not appropriately diagnosed, the results will be less than satisfactory.

RSD

This syndrome is the most elusive nerve problem of the foot and leg to diagnose and is the least understood. There are other names for RSD like causalgia, Sudek's atrophy, and shoulder-hand syndrome. It involves the autonomic nervous system.

RSD usually occurs after a variety of minor (ankle sprain) or major (crush, fracture, or laceration) injuries. It may be related to heart attacks, head trauma, and tumors, or to nothing at all. It occurs more frequently in the shoulder and hand than in the leg and foot. The disease can affect all ages, from children of ten with a simple ankle sprain to the elderly. It appears most commonly in the forty to sixty age population. Teenage girls seem to experience RSD more frequently than boys. The younger the sufferer, the more quickly the disease subsides. There also appears to be a relationship to the patient's psychological state; stress is a factor. Even when it is correctly diagnosed and promptly treated, RSD does not improve quickly or dramatically. Some permanent problems, however, may be avoided with early treatment.

elen is a sixty-four-year-old woman with chronic aching pain in her foot. She had seen several doctors for her problem and had been treated with NSAIDs and physical therapy which included ultrasound. These treatments brought her minimal relief. She had been fitted with plastic arch supports to help her flat foot condition, but these supports caused her more pain and some numbness.

During her examination, I put pressure just behind the inside of her ankle joint and also tapped on the area. This caused a tingling sensation that radiated into the bottom of her foot toward her toes. She had a flat foot with a collapsed arch that was putting more tension and a pulling force on the inside of her foot and on the nerves located there.

I sent her for EMG and Nerve Conduction testing. The results showed abnormalities behind her ankle with the nerve being compressed inside the tarsal tunnel. Since all conservative treatments had failed, Helen elected to have surgery to free the nerve from the constricting tunnel. Her post-operative recovery was slow, but she continued to improve. She had some numbness on the bottom of her foot, but this gradually cleared. She experienced some slight continued aching after being active, but continues to be happy with her new-found function.

Note: *The success rate with tarsal tunnel surgery is variable. It should be used after medical treatment has proven unsuccessful.*

Symptoms

There are three somewhat overlapping stages with symptoms in this disease. The most significant symptom is PAIN out of proportion in severity and length of time to the injury which started it. This is a big part of the index of suspicion in diagnosing RSD. The three stages are:

STAGE	DURATION	SYMPTOMS
1	2-3 months	• Localized severe pain • Burning, tingling, numbness like other nerve problems • Generalized swelling • Pale or mottled skin • Increased warmth in the foot and ankle
2	3-6 months after injury.	• Increased stiffness of the joints • More diffuse pain • Leg soft tissue and muscle atrophy • Osteoporosis changes seen on x-ray
3	6 months to various durations.	• Irreversible changes like permanent joint stiffness, soft tissue, muscle atrophy, and so on. • Generalized leg pain symptoms • Cool, dry, pale, and tense feeling in foot

It is important to recognize these symptoms developing and to see your doctor quickly. Perform gentle exercise to keep joints limber. They include stretching and twisting your toes in a clockwise and then counter-clockwise motion. Using your legs is also necessary.

Self-Help, Medical, and Surgical Treatment

Self-help focuses on simple exercises and the use of mild anti-inflammatory medicine (aspirin, Motrin). However, if pain is significant, early medical help is needed. Early medical diagnosis and treatment may include epidural or sympathetic nerve block injections into the back area, usually given in a series over several weeks. These injections may dramatically relieve the symptoms. Physical therapy to keep limber even if the exercise causes some discomfort helps avoid permanent contractures.

A bone scan can assist the diagnosis of RSD. In this procedure, dye is injected which circulates to areas of active changes in bone and soft tissue. These areas light up as problem areas.

J. P., a thirty-year-old computer scientist, tripped on the stairs at his home and twisted his right ankle rather severely. He had no previous ankle injuries and experienced swelling and pain on the outside of his ankle. He went to the local hospital emergency room. His x-rays showed no fracture. He was treated with ankle immobilization in an air cast and told to use ice, crutches, and NSAIDs. His doctor had put him on a course of physical therapy and had tried a variety of ankle braces.

He came to my office complaining of severe ankle pain that was throughout the foot and not well localized. His ankle was stiff and he had limited function out of proportion to his injury. His examination revealed a mottled looking foot with generalized swelling. His injured right foot was cold compared to his left, and his joints were tight.

X-rays showed no fractures (broken bones), but the bones showed a loss of calcification (osteoporosis). His pain symptoms were more severe than the injury warranted and, with the bone changes, I made a preliminary diagnosis of RSD. I sent him for a bone scan which showed increased circulation to all areas of the foot.

He was treated with a series of three epidural back injections to anesthetize the autonomic nervous system to his foot. He was given the nerve medicine Elavil and was put into an aggressive physical therapy program to include range of motion, strengthening, and progressive weight bearing exercises.

He responded dramatically and continued physical therapy for six weeks. He gradually recovered.

Note: *RSD runs a variable course and is diagnosed as an index of suspicion. It is often missed for some months after the injury. The sooner that aggressive treatment is started, the quicker the patient will begin to recover. Even with proper treatment, some problems from RSD may continue to persist indefinitely.*

If the RSD is stress-related, psychological counseling is recommended. Anti-depressants or nerve medicines like Tegretal may relieve symptoms. As an alternative, steroids can also be injected to provide some relief. There are three other methods of treatment that help RSD sufferers. These are TENS units, ultrasound, and occasionally acupuncture. TENS unit is a low voltage electric stimulus unit which interrupts and treats a pain cycle. There are also RSD support groups that provide counseling, advice, and information about this difficult disease.

Surgery is rarely performed on the affected part since it may result in more nerve damage and disabling pain. If scar tissue or ligament tightness causes nerve compression in the leg and contributes to RSD, surgical release of the tissues and nerve is occasionally attempted. However, the results are *not* predictable. In severe refractory cases, surgical sympathectomy (cutting of the sympathetic nerve ganglia) may be performed in the back region by a general surgeon. Amputation of the leg may be necessary, but even this does not guarantee success.

IN A NUTSHELL

The most common nerve problem you might have in your foot is Morton's neuroma or tarsal tunnel syndrome. However, any nerve can be involved. A classic symptom of a nerve problem is tinel which produces tingling and numbness, radiating away from a nerve up into the foot or leg when you tap on it. Both Morton's neuroma and tarsal tunnel can be treated by proper shoes or metatarsal pads, limiting the offending activities. The final step is performing surgery, if the symptoms continue.

A difficult nerve problem to diagnose and treat is RSD which affects your autonomic nervous system. When your pain is all out of proportion to your injury, RSD is suspected. Early medical treatment is very important. Even then, the recovery time is prolonged.

DOCTOR'S CORNER:
QUESTIONS AND ANSWERS

I have Morton's neuroma tumor and have had a little pain for about six weeks. The pain is much worse after I wear my high heels to work. Should I have surgery?

Morton's neuroma is an inflamed and swollen nerve that passes under the ball of the foot. It isn't a tumor, although it can be very troublesome and even disabling. This condition is aggravated by high heels and pointed toe shoes, because this type of shoe compresses the metatarsal bones.

First, stop wearing these shoes and find wider toe box, lower heel shoes to quiet down your inflammation. You can also try NSAIDS and metatarsal pads to spread your metatarsal bones a little to help relieve pressure. Your doctor can also inject the area with anesthetic and cortisone to try to relieve painful symptoms.

If your symptoms still worsen after all these treatments have failed, then surgery to remove the neuroma should be considered. There is about seventy-five percent chance of success in achieving a dramatic relief of pain, but it is important for you to remember that the nerve is actually cut and there is always risk that a new neuroma will form. This may need repeated surgery to cut the nerve at a different location.

My doctor says that I have a compressed posterior tibial nerve that needs surgery. What should I expect from this surgery?

Tarsal tunnel nerve problems are extremely difficult to diagnose. The electricity test may be normal or inconclusive. So the diagnosis is based on a careful history by examination (especially tinel), and on the index of suspicion.

Results from tarsal tunnel surgery and other nerve surgery is harder to predict than other foot surgery. In most cases, it should be done after other conservative measures have been tried and failed. If tarsal tunnel is the confirmed correct diagnosis, its cause needs to be determined. An MRI will usually help locate any fatty tumor or other cause. Surgery will release the ligament that forms a tunnel for the nerve and the nerve itself is freed and explored for problems.

After surgery, some numbness may persist, but usually improves over the next few months. The pain relief should be dramatic. Some surgeons report a success rate of seventy-five percent and others report a little less. Of course, like any surgery, nerve surgery is not guaranteed. It is possible to have little or no improvement. In rare cases, the condition might be made worse.

TERMS TO REMEMBER

Causalgia syndrome: See RSD.

EMG: Electro Myographic study to diagnose muscle function abnormality, electrically using electrodes on the skin or fine gauge needles in the muscle.

Epidural anesthesia: Injection of the back around the sympathetic nerve origins (ganglia) with nerve-numbing and cortisone-type medicines. May not have a lasting effect.

Interdigital neuroma: See Morton's neuroma.

Lipoma: A benign over-growth of fatty tissue.

Morton's neuroma: Interdigital neuroma; pain on the bottom of the foot under the pad of the third or fourth toe—occasionally between the second and third toe.

Nerve Conduction Velocity: An electrical study which measures the speed of nerve conduction to help diagnose nerve abnormalities; not painful and not risky.

Neurologist: A medical doctor specializing in all forms of nerve disease and problems often trained in EMG and Nerve Conduction studies.

Neuroma: A swelling of a nerve associated with inflammation of the nerve or the tissue surrounding the nerve.

Physiatrist: A medical doctor specializing in non-operative muscle and skeletal conditions and trained to perform EMG and nerve conduction studies.

RSD: Reflex sympathetic dystrophy; causalgia (pain) syndrome.

Tarsal tunnel: The tunnel formed by ligaments tissue through which the major foot nerves run. It is located on the inside (medial) side of the ankle area.

TENS unit: A low voltage electric stimulus unit which interrupts and treats a pain cycle.

Tinel: Direct pressure or tapping of a painful nerve area causes tingling and numbness which radiates away from the nerve, usually into the foot and toes, but occasionally backward up into the leg.

CHAPTER 8

My Heels Are Killing Me. What Can I Do?

Time wounds all heels

—JANE ACE, Goodman Ace; *The Fine Art of Hypochondria; Or, How Are You?*

INTRODUCTION

Over the years, the poor heel has acquired a bad name. A heel is known to be a despicable person with a lack of decency or honor. Contrary to such beliefs, a heel is a productive part of the human anatomy. It has durable shock absorbing qualities that cushion the day-to-day pounding

Dealing with heel pain and related problems requires patience. They are annoying, but treatable. Start with self-help and then see if you need medical treatment or surgery.

it takes. It is also critical to one's gait. You can see why it is so important to keep the heel healthy at all times.

"*My heel hurts,*" is one of the most common complaints I hear in my busy orthopedic foot clinic. This annoying symptom has generally been a problem for my patients for several months before they seek medical attention. Heel pain is not easy to treat and healing time is prolonged since we need to walk on our feet.

Heel pain and heel problems in general are the result of overstressing the heel bone or walking on hard surfaces such as concrete sidewalks for a prolonged period. Sooner or later, the tissue that pads the bone begins to wear away, causing heel pain. The first sign is usually a mild heel pain with a feeling of discomfort like a heel bruise. Eventually, the arch of the foot begins to hurt. It is a potentially debilitating problem.

There are many reasons for feeling pain in the heel. In this chapter, the focus is on heel pain and its many ramifications—its causes, treatment, and how to avoid such discomfort. Remember that heel pain is essentially an inflammation of the tissue that covers the heel bone. Repeated stress or injury causes the inflammation that signals the pain.

NATURAL HISTORY

Heel pain spares no one. It can begin at any age, although it characteristically appears for the first time in middle age. It is more common in people with heavier builds and often starts gradually for no obvious reason. The heel pain is aggravated by weight bearing. It is consistently worse when you first get up in the morning and at the end of the day. The pain usually lurks in the heel pad and may include the arch ligament. Since some aching is associated with middle age, there is a tendency to ignore the heel pain at first. Most people follow a pattern of easing up on activities, hoping the pain will go away. This brings to mind the five most common words in medicine, "Maybe it will go away!"

For many patients with heel pain, it all begins when they commit to a new physical activity after a period of relative inactivity. One or both heels may be symptomatic, although one usually hurts more than the other. If heel pain is left untreated, it may gradually abate and even clear up altogether in nine to twelve months. Even with treatment, the patient needs patience! Heel pain requires a prolonged period of recovery and can be frustrating for both patient and doctor.

HEEL ANATOMY AND ASSOCIATED PAIN

There are several components of the heel anatomy that contribute to the "heel pain syndrome":

- Heel pad or cushion

- Heel bone (os calcis) and heel spur

- Arch ligament (plantar fascia)

- Heel cord (Achilles tendon)

- The nerve to the small muscles of the foot that pass behind the ankle (tarsal tunnel). See figure 8-1 for nerves in the heel and heel anatomy.

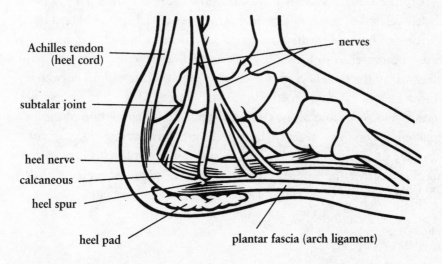

FIGURE 8-1. *Nerves in the heel and heel anatomy*

As one ages, soft tissues become more worn and the heel pad cushions (fatty cushion layer) become thinner and less shock absorbent. In middle age, the forefoot tends to spread because of increasing stretching of forefoot ligaments. As a result, you can expect some collapse of the arch itself. If you are in this age group, your arches will collapse more and more, causing additional stress on our arch ligaments. When this happens, "microtears" occur where the arch ligament attaches to the heel. In this area, a small bony spur is often identified.

Heel pain patients usually have tight and inflexible heel cords or what we call Achilles tendon tightness. When the heel cord is tight, it causes us to compensate by overpronating our feet for proper foot weight bearing. Sometimes Achilles tendinitis causes heel pain. A more detailed discussion of this problem is covered in chapter 12.

A typical heel pain patient has either a high arch (pes cavus) with a very tight arch ligament or a flat foot appearance (pes planus). There may be some associated tingling or numbness that radiates to the bottom of the foot toward the big toe, small toe, or even the outside and bottom of the heel. These symptoms may be secondary to tight ligaments behind the ankle which could result in Tarsal tunnel symptoms. (See chapter 7). Other possibilities are secondary symptoms from compression or irritation of the heel nerve that passes directly under the heel. This nerve is closely related to the arch ligament attachment, heel spur, and heel bone.

A small heel spur (often only a few millimeters in size) can be identified on the heel from foot x-rays. It seems like the culprit for heel pain, but most of the time heel spur is only an incidental finding. The arch ligament attaches directly to this immediate area. Most doctors feel heel spur develops because of the continual pull and inflammation of the arch ligament. Foot x-rays usually show heel spurs on both feet, although only one may be painful. Most likely, the culprit is the entire heel bone striking into the heel pad during the "heel strike" phase of walking. If left untreated, it can eventually cause heel pad damage and pain.

Associated Causes and Treatments

There are several causes of heel pain. Here are four major causes:

- Prolonged standing promotes the kind of stress that could inflame the heel.

- Obesity—carrying "extra baggage"—is the cause of all sorts of foot problems, especially heel pain. It contributes to a disproportionate pressure (and discomfort) to both feet.

- Previous serious foot or heel injury or repeated injury from virtually any other causes.

- Running, jogging, or fast walking, especially when you are not conditioned for such high energy exercise.

There are also several associated symptoms of heel pain:

- Heel cushion pain. The thin heel pad may become painful in examination when pressed upon and the heel bone can be felt.

- Tingling or numbness of the bottom (sole or plantar side) of the foot.

- Tight and painful arch ligament (plantar fascia) made worse by rolling over the ball of the foot. Normally, this walking action tightens, stresses, and stabilizes the ligament.

- Heel cord swelling and pain (Achilles tendinitis).

- Metatarsalgia and claw toes from the associated high arch.

- Recurrent shin splints history. This suggests hyper-pronation or a flat foot stress problem.

Following are other diseases associated with heel and ankle pain. All of these diseases should be treated medically (see chapter 11):

- Plantar fibromatosis
- Ankylosing spondylitis
- Reiter's syndrome
- Psoriasis
- Lyme disease
- Rheumatoid arthritis
- Gout
- Colitis

It is important to recognize these symptoms and check with your doctor accordingly. Preventive steps can save a lot of discomfort and unnecessary pain for patient and family.

Self-Treatment

Here are some ideas that can help you weather the pain:

- If you are heavy, lose weight! It is not an easy task. Take this step in stages and consult your doctor for proper nourishment and exercise.

- Provide better heel cushioning by using cup or soft heel cushion shoe inserts. Try to pad the bottom of the heel to take the stress off the spot where the pain is. This pad goes directly inside the shoe.

- Wear soft-soled shoes. This can make a major impact (no pun intended) on your heel.

- Use a soft arch-foot support like Spenko or Dr. Scholl's to cushion the heel and support your arch.

- Try a plastic heel cup which may stabilize your heel pad a bit and provide better shock absorption. See figure 8-2.

- Gently stretch your heel and arch ligament before you get out of bed in the morning. This should be followed by a warm soak in the tub or shower followed by more stretching. Do the stretching slowly. If you feel burning in the back of the leg or bottom of the feet, you may be stretching too far and should ease off a bit. Stretch your heels before you get out of bed and before you rise from sitting for an extended period of time. The heel stretch involves pointing your toes toward your nose. You may do one or both legs at a time. To be effective, this stretch must be held for at least fifteen seconds and needs to be repeated three times a day. If done properly, this stretch is the simplest and most effective treatment for heel pain. You should consider making it a part of your daily life, since heel pain tends to recur. DON'T EXPECT IMMEDIATE RESULTS. Long-term gain is the goal. See chapter 12 on exercise and proper stretching techniques for more details.

- When you first have pain, use ice on your heels for fifteen to twenty minutes twice a day. Repeat the ice treatment at least two more times during the day for the same time period.

- Try aspirin or NSAIDs two to three times a day, or as prescribed. Be aware of side effects. Don't use these medicines if you have any stomach problems. Always check with your doctor if you are taking other potentially conflicting medicine.

- Be aware of activities that aggravate the heel pain problem and avoid ill-fitting shoes, wrong exercises, and overstress. A word to the wise—don't do too much too soon in your exercise/conditioning program.

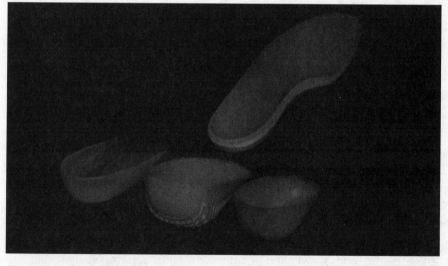

FIGURE 8-2. *Variety of heel cushions*

Medical Treatment

After you have gone the self-help route, if symptoms of heel pain persist, go to your foot specialist for professional treatment. The longer you wait for help, the longer chronic inflammation and pain will persist even after treatment has taken place. As a routine procedure, x-rays are taken to identify unusual causes of heel pain such as arthritis, stress, fractures, or bony tumors.

Occasionally, heel pain is associated with a systemic disease like Reiter's disease, a viral disease often including eye inflammation, genital discharge, and/or back and stomach problems. It can also be a symptom of colitis (a bowel inflammation), ankylosing spondylitis (stiff back arthritis), rheumatoid arthritis, or systemic lupus erythematosis. These diseases require specialized blood tests, x-rays, and diagnostic studies for appropriate diagnoses.

For refractory (resistent) heel pain symptoms, custom fabricated orthotics may be needed to control pronation, provide support, and aid cushioning. Sometimes, a semi-rigid (plastic) device is used, but an accommodative cushion support is more common.

Physical therapy is often prescribed for two to three weeks to ensure the heel pain patient uses proper stretching techniques. The therapist can also treat the soft tissue with a variety of soft tissue modalities including massage, cryotherapy (cold treatment), or ultrasound (deep heat). Occasionally, ionophoresis or cortisone ointment is applied to counteract inflammation. Taping or velcro strapping the arch may also be used in an attempt to relieve the stress area. See taping technique in chapter 16.

If your symptoms are severe enough or persist in spite of the other treatments, then your doctor may inject a certain dosage of cortisone and Xylocaine (a form of Novocaine) into your heel. A series of two to three injections may be performed over several weeks in an attempt to get lasting relief. Remember that injections without proper stretching exercises and cushioning devices are not recommended. Also, repeated injections of cortisone tends to weaken ligaments and joints, particularly if they are repeated excessively. Adverse reaction to the cortisone ingredients occurs

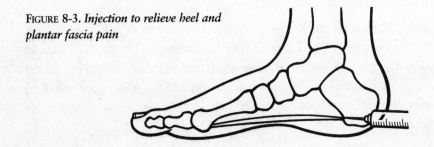

FIGURE 8-3. *Injection to relieve heel and plantar fascia pain*

in 6 to 10 percent of patients. It is manifested by pain and worsening of their symptoms for six to twenty-four hours. This is nothing serious, as it will correct spontaneously and treatment is the use of ice, NSAIDs, and pain medicine. See figure 8-3.

A more recent treatment that I use for persistent heel pain is a night cast which provides more prolonged stretching of the heel cord and arch ligaments while the patient is asleep. A trained cast technician makes a special removable brace or cast. The patient wears the device for two to three hours at first and then gradually increases the time until it can be worn comfortably all night. Many resistent cases of heel pain and arch ligament pain have been significantly helped by this type of night cast.

Surgical Treatment

When proper medical and self-help treatment fails and non-improving symptoms persist over eight to twelve months, then surgery is recommended. Since heel pain takes a year or so to heal, there should be no rush into surgery. The surgery performed depends on the anatomical structures which might include the following:

- *Arch ligament release*—this ligament is released partially or completely where it inserts into the heel.

- *Release of the tight inside muscle and nerve* in its tunnel if nerve symptoms are present.

- *Removal of the heel spur*—It is rarely done, unless the spur is large.

- *Endoscopic* or small incision techniques can be used to release the ligament. Since this technique is still being developed, make sure your surgeon has experience using this procedure. It only has limited application and cannot be used to relieve the entrapped nerve, the tight foot muscle or, if the spur is large enough, to remove the heel spur.

Expectations and Complications

If the ligament has been released, a slightly more flattened arch may result. This rarely is a problem, but could lead to some flat foot strain requiring further treatment. Occasional numbness may occur if one of the heel nerves is accidentally stretched or injured. Some numbness may linger after releasing the heel nerve, but usually this will resolve itself with time.

Casting, splints, and/or crutches are used after surgery for several weeks with gradual resumption of weight bearing when healing has occurred. Gentle physical therapy is recommended for proper stretching techniques. Proper shoes and supports are also important. The success rate with heel surgery is about eighty percent.

In summary, dealing with heel pain and related problems means *patience*. It can be annoying and discomforting, but it is treatable. If you heed the symptoms and follow the self-help steps, you should get better. Of course, you can and should consult your doctor if symptoms persist.

OTHER CAUSES OF PLANTAR (ARCH LIGAMENT) PAIN

Plantar Fibromatosis

This problem is a localized excess growth of the arch ligament. It assumes a nodular appearance, and the cause is unknown. The condition is frequently painful and often enlarges, but it is not cancer. Similar nodules can appear in the hand which cause a contraction of the fingers called *Dupuytren's Contracture*.

Plantar Nodule

If the plantar thickening is painless and is not becoming larger, it is best left alone. However, it should periodically be checked by a doctor. If symptoms or enlargement occurs, wide surgical removal of the ligament and growth is required. Occasionally, skin healing problems or even some foot numbness may occur after this type of surgery. See figure 8-4.

Foot Tumors

Any growth or lump in the foot should be evaluated by a foot specialist. Fortunately, cancers to the foot's soft tissue or bone are extremely rare. Increasing pain or ulceration with a failure to heal should be medically evaluated.

Nancy, a forty-five-year-old woman, had gained over twenty pounds over the past few years. In an attempt to lose this weight, she began a walking program. She wore tennis shoes for the exercise. She gradually increased her distance and speed but began to have aching in the heel pad area of her foot. She continued walking for another month. The pain increased, especially early in the walking program and began to interfere with other daily activities. Stiffness and pain were troublesome in the early morning but subsided some after Nancy was up and active. She stopped her program for over three weeks and became rather inactive, hoping that the rest would cure her heel pain.

After three weeks, she resumed her program and the symptoms returned. She was frustrated and a friend told her she probably had a heel spur. She came to my office and, upon examination, I found tenderness when her heel was pushed. The heel pad was not firm. She had slight tenderness on the arch ligament and felt pain there when her toes were bent upward. She had tight heel cords and pronated slightly. X-rays were normal but showed a small insignificant heel spur.

Nancy was treated with heel cushions, a Spenko arch support, NSAIDS, moist morning soaks and ice massage during the day. She started physical therapy for heel cord and plantar fascia stretching. Prestretching her heel cord and plantar fascia before getting out of bed was emphasized. She was advised to get good walking shoes with cushioned supportive soles and heels. Her symptoms improved gradually over the next month. She had a heel injection of cortisone and anesthetics which gave her added relief. She gradually resumed her walking program and slowly increased the speed and distance. She was encouraged to continue to lose weight. She still experiences some mild aching but has resumed all her normal activities.

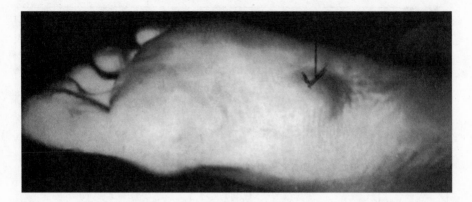

FIGURE 8-4. *Plantar nodule*

IN A NUTSHELL

Heel pain appears in middle age, but can be a problem for all ages. It often shows up when you start a new activity like an exercise program, especially in overweight people. It can also be associated with an inflamed arch ligament (plantar fascia), a weakening of the heel pad, or a combination of these. Rarely, the heel nerve is irritated. Heel spurs sound like the culprits causing heel pain, but in most cases, they are unrelated to the problem. Heel pain is often ignored until it becomes severe and disabling. It is a difficult problem to treat and requires a prolonged recovery. Patience is critical.

DOCTOR'S CORNER:
QUESTIONS AND ANSWERS

My doctor advised me to have night casts made for my heel pain. They seem like such a nuisance. Are they worth the trouble?

Night casting is a way to stretch the foot and ankle ligaments. The goal is to relieve heel pain. Increasing foot flexibility is key and night casts seem to help. I suggest that other stretching exercises be performed several times a day.

If heel problems persist, often dramatic help can come with night casts. It is important to allow your body to adjust to wearing these casts. Start out wearing them for a short period of time and increase the time when some flexibility is gained. The same thing applies to wearing new orthotics.

I had an injection of cortisone in my heel and it helped the pain for several weeks. How often can I have these shots?

If heel pain symptoms are severe and disabling, injecting the heel will often give pain relief and allows better stretching exercises to be performed. These exercises are very important. I will only repeat injections twice more over a period of several months. The goal is to obtain more lasting relief. Cortisone injections have a tradeoff. They are excellent anti-inflammatory medicines, but they cause weakening of the ligaments and atrophy of the heel pad. Therefore, this treatment should not be used too many times. Most heel pain syndrome problems gradually get better over six months to a year.

TERMS TO REMEMBER

Arch ligament (plantar fascia): A band of strong fibers or the ligament that connects the heel to the toes and runs along the arch of the foot.

Colitis: A bowel inflammation.

Contusion: A bruising injury that does not break the skin.

Foot tumor: Can involve the skin, soft tissue (lump), or bone. It is frequently, though not always, associated with pain, and it is rarely cancer. You should consult your doctor for an evaluation.

Heel bone: The os calcis or calcaneous bone. It is the largest foot bone.

Heel cord (Achilles tendon): The large tendon in the back of the ankle.

Heel pad: The soft tissue of the heel, primarily made up of fatty tissue. It is the primary shock absorber.

Heel pain syndrome: Localized or central heel pad tenderness which is the most frequent cause of heel pain.

Heel spur: An edge of bone that juts out of the heel bone. It usually is not the cause of the pain.

Orthotics: Molded or standard inserts which are placed inside the shoe.

Plantar fibromatosis: A benign nodular thickening of the arch ligament.

Spur: A bony outgrowth.

Ultrasound: A physical therapy technique that uses heat from high frequency sound waves to break up scar tissue, increasing circulation and reducing swelling.

CHAPTER 9

Is There a Treatment for Flat Feet?

INTRODUCTION

This chapter is about flat feet and pronation. It is one type of deviation not found in the normal foot. A normal foot conforms to four criteria: The arch is not too flat or too high, no problem calluses are present, the toes are straight, and there is no foot pain.

People with flat feet have minimal or no arch in the foot and the arch lies flat against the floor. Having a flat foot is a foot posture and may cause a variety of problem symptoms for some people. Other lucky folks

Having flat feet can be a problem. With or without pain, they can cause bunions and impingement of the ankle ligaments, tendons, and nerves. Check with your doctor, as it is easy to mistake flat foot tendon rupture deformity as an ankle sprain.

with flat feet have no symptoms at all. Associated with flat feet is pronation or a functional rolling inward of the foot while walking or running. This results in a twisting effect on the whole leg. Some people who walk with excessive pronation, however, do not have flat feet. In this chapter, we refer to pronation as a function and a flat foot as a foot posture. See figure 9-1.

NATURAL HISTORY

The natural history of the flat foot is poorly understood. As in most foot problems, flat feet may display a myriad of symptoms for the patient, or none at all. This condition may start at any age and has an unpredictable natural history. It is important to note that in infancy and early childhood, the foot normally appears flat. The bones of the foot are not fully developed and continue to mature until about age fifteen. The fatty tissue around the arch makes it look flat. The foot muscles are not developed until the child has been standing and walking for a few years. By age ten, the basic foot structure has formed.

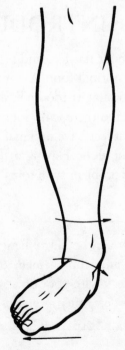

FIGURE 9-1. *Standing flat foot (posture) Pronation (function showing rolling over of the flat in walking)*

During the early walking phase, restrictive shoes should not be worn as they only delay normal muscle development. Between ages three and six, the normal child is knock-kneed which causes pressure on the inside of the foot. It results in a "normal" flat foot during the growth phase. It appears at its worst angulation at age three or four. But by age five or six, the leg straightens and the arch assumes the less flat adult appearance.

THE FLEXIBLE FLAT FOOT

The *flexible flat foot* is the one most commonly seen. It has a typical form. While the person is sitting, the arch appears normal, but flattens when standing. See figure 9-2. There are no statistics as to prevalence. It seems more common in infants and children, and resolves spontaneously in the majority of cases. Most children and adolescents with this condition don't complain of foot symptoms and generally lead very active lives. They may have an occasional arch ache but rarely require medical treatment for the condition.

A small percentage of children have symptoms in their early years. This group usually has a bony abnormality in the arch (**accessory navicular**) which appears as a prominence. A few children have such a significant collapse of the arch that the bones and ligaments in it become deformed. If this condition limits their activities, they may need medical or surgical treatment sometime during their foot development period.

Pronation and the abnormal twisting associated with flat feet in active young athletes may cause shin splints, knee cap and knee problems, hip strain, and back pain. See chapter 12 for details.

Foot research over the past decade suggests that many adults with mild flat feet in their early years are candidates for medical treatment by middle age. They generally state that their feet are getting flatter. These patients tend to be overweight and their foot problems become significantly more serious.

Since the posterior tibia tendon is the major supporting muscle/tendon unit of the arch, rupture of this tendon is a recently recognized cause for worsening of the flat foot in adults. The posterior tibial tendon rupture can be from an injury, but it is important to note that the wear and

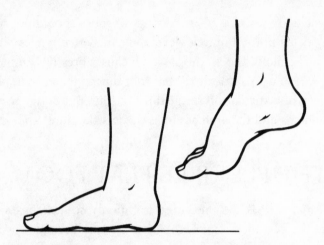

FIGURE 9-2. *Standing flat foot and sitting flat foot. In the flexible flat foot, the arch is restored when sitting (non-weight bearing).*

tear of age can also weaken this tendon. During the middle forties, the problem often worsens. Once the tendon fails, the patient develops arch pain. The deformity and symptoms will continue to progress with age unless the patient seeks medical/surgical treatment.

Symptoms of Flat Feet

A major symptom to watch for is abnormal shoe wear. With flat feet, the patient's shoes have a breakdown on the inside wall of the heel. The inside sole of the shoe is also quickly worn down.

In the rigid flat foot patient, hindfoot joints may be congenitally fused (**tarsal coalition**). They may also be the result of changes due to arthritis or a variety of causes. The rigid flat foot limits the joints' adaptability to walk on uneven surfaces and causes pain and discomfort. The normal shock absorption of the foot is lost. Pain may be transmitted to other areas like the leg, knee, or back. While standing, the rigid flat foot looks just like the flexible flat foot.

In some people with flat feet, a large bump on the arch area (accessory navicular bone) is present from birth. They usually display no symptoms, but may have some excess pressure felt from their shoes. Strain on the legs with microtears in the arch is often caused by chronic stress. The arch becomes inflamed and aches. The pain worsens after activity and

R ose, a forty-three-year-old design consultant, came to our clinic four months after her ankle injury. She had been treated by her family physician for an ankle sprain. Her symptoms were swelling and pain on the inside of her ankle that had persisted long beyond the normal healing time for her injury. She had bilateral flat feet and had never been treated for this condition. She had noticed an increased flattening of her foot after her injury.

At examination, she displayed swelling and pain on the inside of her ankle. Typical ankle sprains display pain and swelling on the outside of the ankle. An MRI was ordered. It confirmed the diagnosis of a ruptured posterior tibia tendon. This is the major supporting muscle/tendon group of the arch. Surgery was performed to stabilize the bones around her arch to prevent further foot deformity.

Rose has recovered and once again leads a very busy, active life.

that's when the inflammation is greatest. The flat foot of such a patient has loose ligaments, but the Achilles tendon (heel cord) is very tight. The foot is attached to the ankle which is attached to the leg. So the body compensates for this condition by straining the foot joints while searching for flexibility. The strain contributes to the development of a flatter foot.

People with excessive pronation are forced to place more stress on the big toe. Bunions develop or existing ones get worse. As the big toe loses flexibility, it transfers stresses, and calluses develop on the ball (**plantar pads**) of the foot. As the flat foot progresses, the heel angles out more instead of being straight. Gradually, the outside of the ankle will become painful as ligaments and tendons are pinched (**impingement syndrome**) by the collapse of the heel bones against the ankle bones. This deformity gets worse. Eventually, the joints will dislocate and become inflexible. Arthritis of the hindfoot joints develops and causes a general, aching pain.

Remember, the twisting effect of a flat foot deformity puts abnormal torque (rotational) stress on the knee, hip, and back. The major symptoms displayed are pain and discomfort in these areas instead of in the foot itself. This is particularly true if the patient has a pre-existing knee,

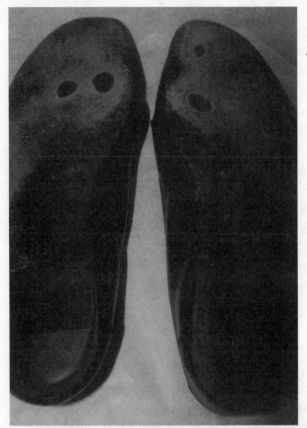

FIGURE 9-3. *Shoe wear patterns*

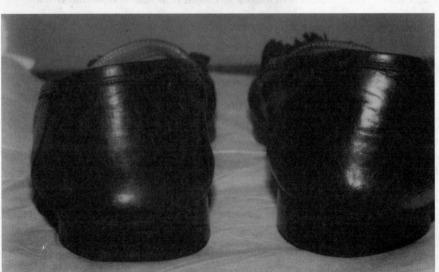

hip, or back disc problem. The reverse is also true where patients with knee arthritis may develop flat feet because of the bowing out stress of the knees.

Evaluating shoe wear is quite helpful in appreciating the magnitude of flat foot deformity. The inside sole of the shoe is quickly worn down and the outer part of the heel often is excessively worn, as well. For example, the foot strikes on the outside heel and quickly and excessively rolls to the inside foot (pronation).

Summary

To summarize, flat feet display several problem symptoms:

- Inside arch ligament strain and ache
- Inside the ankle swelling
- Bunion symptoms (see chapter 5)
- Outside ankle pain (impingement syndrome)
- Rigid foot—no shock absorption
- Arthritis—foot, ankle, toe joints
- Shin-splints, knee pain, back pain

Self-Help Treatment

If the patient is overweight, losing weight is a welcome relief for the flat foot. Remember, pressure relates to pounds per square inch. Heel cord (Achilles tendon) stretching exercises are used to gain flexibility and relieve arch ligament and tendon stress. Simple stretching is recommended two or three times a day, although one should not expect immediate improvement. Yet, the long-term benefit is relief of pain and discomfort. Stretching along with strengthening the posterior tibia muscle is the most beneficial treatment you can do for yourself. See chapter 15. Arch supports and good supporting shoes with arch inserts are also helpful.

Medical Treatment

There is no evidence to show that shoe modifications make much difference in the natural history of the flexible flat foot. These modifications might make the foot "look better" and extend shoe life. But they can help relieve the foot arch pain with no change in the flat foot.

Nonsteroidal arthritis medicine may reduce the pain, swelling, and arthritis aching symptoms related to flat feet. There are also other treatments:

- Warm foot soaks

- Ice to help reduce swelling

- Physical therapy with modalities like ultrasound

- Stretching and strengthening exercises to stretch tight heel cords and plantar fascia

- Steroid cream (iontophoresis-phonophoreses)

- Home exercise programs

- Inside (medial) heel or sole wedges in the shoe

Custom-molded orthotics and/or arch support use special casting techniques to help relieve symptoms. This treatment is especially important during the foot development years and in older patients where health conditions eliminate surgery as an option. Remember that custom orthotics need proper shoes to work right. Orthotics are expensive and may only last from one to two years. Unfortunately, many insurance programs do not cover their cost. Orthotics also do *not* always work! A short-leg brace, from the foot to just below the knee that has the proper shoe support, occasionally limits foot stress and provides the patient with some shock absorption.

Surgical Treatment

Flat feet, particularly in adult onset, is a progressive problem. Surgery is frequently indicated to halt the deformity caused by this condition. Surgery may be recommended either to stabilize the primary flat foot problem or to treat associated symptoms, especially bunions. Any surgical procedure *must* be followed by proper shoes and supports.

The most common surgical procedures performed for flat feet patients are:

1. Tendon transfers and ligament tightening procedures to provide more soft tissue and bony support.

2. Arthrodesis (fusion) of the hindfoot joints which may require the use of bone grafts from the pelvis or leg bones to aid in healing.

3. Lengthening or loosening of the tight heel cord (Achilles tendon).

4. Osteotomies (cutting) of the heel (os calcis) or foot bones to change the flat foot angle. This procedure is primarily considered for the child, adolescent, or young adult patient.

Surgical Expectations and Complications

Any surgery is major, requiring a few days of hospitalization to adequately control pain and swelling. Usually, pain decreases markedly each day. Casting is generally required for two to three months. Crutches are also used and the surgical foot is restricted in weight bearing for the first six weeks. A progressive weight bearing/walking program is prescribed for the next six weeks. Remember that if the operated foot is your driving foot, you will be unable to drive during the healing/casting period. Screws, pins, wires, and even bone staples are often used for stabilizing the bones. These devices are safe; they have been used by surgeons for many years and are not rejected by the body. They rarely require removal after healing. On occasion, they may rub and cause discomfort, requiring surgical removal. Depending on the location of the device, they can often be removed in your doctor's office or in a minor surgical environment. This second surgery rarely involves any significant pain or complications.

All foot surgeries cause foot and ankle swelling. One reason is that the feet are the farthest points of the body from the heart. As a result, swelling may persist for several months rather than weeks. Occasionally, swelling may become a permanent condition. Proper shoes that fit well and arch supports are extremely important to promote healing and prevent recurrence of the problem. Occasionally, pain and/or arthritis may develop in other foot joints as a result of fusing the hindfoot. Fortunately, this develops late in life and is usually mild compared to the original problem. If tendon surgery alone is performed in an attempt to preserve joint flexibility, the newly created tissue supports may not be adequate to do the job. Subsequent fusion may have to be done. In terms of infection, it occurs in one to three percent of surgical cases. In some cases, blood clots may form which require medical treatment with blood thinners and hospitalization.

The most common problem with hindfoot fusion is the failure of the joints to fuse or heal. This may require a second surgery and/or a bone stimulator (electrical stimulation) to ensure proper foot stability. Pain symptoms should continue to diminish during the year after surgery. All or most of the pain symptoms are eventually relieved.

Even though fusion sounds like a drastic approach, most patients end up walking without a noticeable limp and pain disappears after healing takes place. You may lose some ability to adjust to uneven surfaces and you may have to alter your lifestyle accordingly. On the other hand, remember the condition and limiting function you encountered prior to fusion surgery. The major reason for this surgery is pain control.

IN A NUTSHELL

People with flat feet often pronate excessively, which causes them to roll their feet inward while they are walking or running. Flat feet may or may not get progressively worse. Symptoms range from no pain or problems to disabling pain in the arch. They can cause bunions and impingement of the ankle ligaments, tendons, and nerves.

Pay attention to pain if it is of recent onset, especially if you are having pain on the inside of the ankle joint. This is of particular importance if you have a progressive flat foot deformity. It is easy to mistake this condition as an ankle sprain, but it is actually a failure or rupture of the posterior tibial tendon which supports the arch. This specific flat foot problem begins in adulthood, often requiring surgery to repair the tendon and provide better support for the arch.

DOCTOR'S CORNER:
QUESTIONS AND ANSWERS

My child is ten and has very flat feet which don't seem to bother him. Should I do anything about this?

If your child has no symptoms or associated problems with his flat feet, there are no specific medical treatments that are necessary. Simple arch supports or even molded orthotics help painful arch conditions if they develop. But there is no supporting evidence that using them will help create a better arch.

I do recommend stretching the heel cords for people with flat feet, because their Achilles tendons are tight. Your child needs to learn the proper stretching techniques and needs to do these exercises regularly to help take some pressure off his arch. This will help his condition.

I am fifty-five and in good health. My orthopedic doctor diagnosed my ruptured posterior tibial tendon and recommends repairing it, then using another tendon to lift my arch. He also recommends cutting my heel bone. What should I expect? Do I have any other choices?

In patients who are young to middle age and not excessively overweight, a surgical attempt to restore a supporting ankle structure and change the angle of the heel by osteotomy is appropriate if the foot is flexible and has no apparent arthritis. The goal is to relieve pain by reinforcing the arch area.

After surgery, the patient is in a series of casts for eight to twelve weeks. A physical therapy rehab program is next and shoe supports will be prescribed. You shouldn't expect a normal-appearing arch, but you have an excellent chance of pain relief and walking comfortably.

If you are very overweight and have a stiff foot or arthritis, you should consider a fusion procedure as a better choice. The pain and deforming condition will be relieved, but you will have some stiffness and may have some difficulty walking on uneven surfaces.

TERMS TO REMEMBER

Accessory navicular: The enlarged anatomical variation of the navicular bone which appears as a bony prominence in the arch. The posterior tibial tendon attaches here.

Achilles tendon: The heel cord which is an extension of the calf muscle and controls the ability to rise on the toes.

Arthrodesis (fusion): The elimination of a specific joint or foot motion by locking bones together to gain stabilization and to eliminate pain.

Flat foot: A foot that lacks or has a decreased arch.

Impingement syndrome: The compression, pinching, and/or irritation of soft tissue—like tendons and ligaments that are under a bony prominence or protrusion.

Os calcis: The heel bone.

Osteotomies: The surgical cutting of bone for realignment and the relief of abnormal pressures causing deformities.

Plantar pad: The fatty tissue on the ball of the foot which acts as a shock absorber.

Posterior tibial muscle/tendon unit: This is the main supporting muscle/tendon unit of the arch. It is located on the inside of the ankle and foot. Shin splints are related to this leg muscle/tendon.

Tarsal coalition: A congenital fusion of two of the mid-tarsal bones of the foot. It is often associated with flat feet and becomes symptomatic in adolescence or young adulthood.

Torque: A twisting force.

PART IV

Problems of All Ages

CHAPTER 10

As a Diabetic, What Do I Need to Know About Diabetes and My Feet?

Man may be the captain of his fate
but he is also the victim of his blood sugar.

—WILFRID G. OAKLEY, *Transactions of the Medical Society of London*, 1962

Diabetes can affect all areas of the body. You need a great deal of knowledge about this disease to avoid serious complications. With today's insulin and proper diet, diabetic persons can now lead a normal life.

INTRODUCTION

Diabetes (diabetes mellitus) is a metabolic disorder caused by the body's inability to transport sugar from blood to cells. The diabetic cannot produce or effectively use insulin, the hormone produced by the pancreas which is necessary for proper sugar utilization. Diabetic patients also tend to suffer from circulatory problems and nerve damage that makes them less sensitive to pain.

Before insulin was discovered in the 1920s, diabetic sufferers did not live very long because of the many secondary complications, including heart and kidney disease and infections. With today's insulin and proper diet, people with diabetes can now lead a normal life. It is important to remember that diabetes can only be controlled, not cured. Therefore, it must be treated with the greatest respect.

This chapter is a *must* for diabetics, family members of diabetic patients, and basic care providers who are screening diabetic problems. You need to understand this illness in order to minimize the many complications associated with the disease. Here are some facts to keep in mind:

- Anyone over age thirty, overweight, and/or with a family history of diabetes is at risk.

- Fourteen million people in the United States and 120 million in the world have diabetes.

- Fifty percent of those with the disease are unaware they have it.

- African-Americans and Hispanics are fifty-five percent more susceptible to getting diabetes than others.

- Foot problems associated with diabetes are the third leading reason for hospitalization.

- Diabetes is the fourth leading cause of death in the U.S.

- Diabetes costs $20 billion per year, or five percent of the total health care budget.

- Fifty to seventy percent of nontraumatic amputations occur in diabetic patients. In those who have had amputations, fifty percent will require a second amputation within five years.

- As many as one in six diabetic patients will develop foot ulcers or have foot abnormality.

- Seventy-five percent of diabetics will experience neuropathy during the course of the disease.

- Diabetics have four times the chance of getting vascular disease. By a twenty-year course of the disease, forty-five percent will experience vascular circulation problems.

- Fifteen percent of the population over age sixty-five will have diabetes.

These facts are cited to focus awareness on the seriousness of this disease. No foot problem in the diabetic patient should be taken lightly. Even a toenail infection is a serious lesion. If you or a loved one have diabetes, you need a great deal of knowledge about it. Diligence can help you avoid some of the serious diabetic foot complications that can result in infection, amputation, or even death.

NATURAL HISTORY

Fortunately, most of the foot problems I treat are not systemic (affecting the entire body). They are biomechanical and often cause simple wear and tear on the lower extremities. But everyone can develop systemic disorders which directly or indirectly affect the health of your feet. Diabetes is a systemic disease that may occur at any age, involving almost every organ in the body. Most of these systemic problems affect the foot one way or the other. Here are some examples:

- Diabetic eyesight problems make it very difficult to monitor the foot carefully. Ulcers or infections can become serious very quickly and can lead to amputation.

- Diabetic kidney disease results in fluid retention that can cause leg and foot swelling. In fact, one-quarter of diabetic sufferers develop foot problems due to the disease.

- Associated vascular disease causes a diminished blood supply to the brain which lessens mental acuity. When this takes place, it is difficult to monitor one's own health on a regular basis.

- Poor nutrition and dehydration associated with diabetes can lead to poor wound healing and diminished mental status.

- Peripheral neuropathy causes a myriad of serious problems. Some of these are:

  - Loss of sensation.

  - Sweating which affects proper temperature control and lubrication and can lead to skin dermatitis and infections.

  - Reduction in muscle control which can lead to foot deformities, pressure areas, ulcers, and amputation.

- A poor white blood cell function (anti-infection cells) increases the chance of infection. Other deficient blood cells also promote blood coagulation which can cause blood clots.

- Hypo or hyperglycemia (too low/too high blood sugar) can cause disorientation. This can lead to injury or organ failure.

IMPORTANT KEY WORDS— TEAMWORK, KNOWLEDGE, AND DILIGENCE

There is a psychological tendency to deny that the disease exists or to disregard its seriousness. Doing so means denying proper care for yourself which can lead to disaster. The best approach to diabetes is a *team approach*. The patient, family, friends, and health care providers need to work together to control as many diabetic complications as possible. The medical team may include family physicians, internists, endocrinologists, neurologists, infectious disease physicians, orthopedists, podiatrists, pedorthists (shoe specialists), physical therapists, ophthalmologists (eye doctors), vascular surgeons, and diabetic foot clinicians.

DIABETIC FOOT PROBLEMS

Foot problems are extremely common in diabetic patients. The incidence of these problems increases the longer the patient has the disease. This is especially true with **peripheral neuropathy, Charcot arthropathy,** and vascular disease complications. In some cases, a foot problem is the initial presenting problem of diabetes, leading to the diagnosis of the disease. Controlling blood sugar may help limit the magnitude of these problems, but does not always preclude their development. For example, type I (juvenile diabetes) usually requires insulin injections and tends to develop more complications. In contrast, type II (adult onset) may be controlled with diet or oral insulin which has fewer complications—although the same complications can occur.

The diabetic foot has four main problems:

• Diabetic vascular disease.

• Diabetic peripheral neuropathy.

• Charcot neuropathy.

• Diabetic ulcers and infections.

An examination of each problem follows.

Diabetic Vascular Disease

This involves both the large vessels of the pelvis and thigh and the smaller vessels below the knee, including the feet. In diabetics, both legs and multiple vessels are frequently diseased. It appears at a younger age (forties or less) and progresses more rapidly than other causes of vascular problems.

There are significant risk factors which worsen the problem. They are listed in order of severity.

- Smoking
- Age—increased risk after age forty
- High blood sugar (hyperglycemia)
- High cholesterol and triglycerides
- High blood pressure (hypertension)

Symptoms

The symptoms of diabetic vascular disease are caused by an inadequate blood supply to various body parts. Even though the artery vessel blockage may be in the thigh or pelvis, pain symptoms may be located in the foot or lower leg. This may be due to numerous collateral or extra vessels supplying the pelvis or thigh. The number diminishes significantly as the flow progresses to the foot. Vascular disease can be missed as a result. Symptoms of vascular insufficiency (**ischemia**) may only occur when the person is active (**claudication**), requiring more circulation and oxygen than normal. During a short period of rest, the pain symptoms may be relieved dramatically.

Among the key symptoms of diabetic vascular disease are:

- Intermittent claudication (walking pain).
- Cold feet.
- Rest pain/night pain, which implies a more severe disease.
- No pulses or decreased pulses.
- Blanching (foot turns white or pale) when the leg is elevated. It becomes red (rubor) when the leg hangs down.
- Loss of hair on the foot or toes.
- Shiny appearance and atrophy (thinning) of tissues.
- Thickened nails—often infected with fungus.
- Gangrene (blue colored toe).
- Foot fissures (cracked skin).
- Dry skin.
- Numbness.

- Ulcers that don't heal well and are painful. Ulcers are breaks in the skin that break down underlying tissue and get worse when not treated.

These symptoms require medical evaluation and aggressive treatment and could save your leg.

Peripheral Neuropathy

The neuropathy of diabetes involves the muscles, sensation, and the autonomic nervous system. It also involves the entire foot in contrast to one nerve problem. However, early in the development of the disease, only part of the system may be affected. On occasion, the diabetic may have a compression of one nerve at the tarsal tunnel which must be considered for proper diagnosis. Loss of the protective sensation often leads to the development of infected ulcers and may contribute to subsequent development of Charcot arthropathy.

The loss of sensation or protective pain is the most common cause of diabetic foot problems. This involves the nervous system which (as discussed in chapter 7) is composed of sensory nerves, motor (muscle supply) nerves, and autonomic nerves. Nerve symptoms characteristically

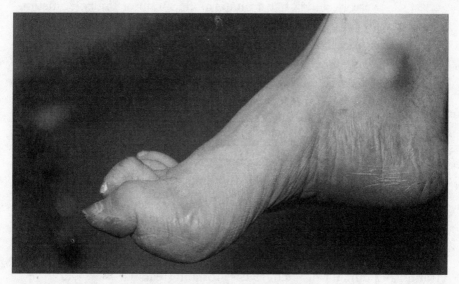

FIGURE 10-1. *Diabetic neuropathy, clawing toes and dry skin*

include night cramps, numbness, tingling, and sometimes radiating pain down the leg. Nerve problems in the diabetic patient are progressive. Seventy-five percent or greater of these people will have neuropathy after twenty years of the disease. The loss of sensation is more severe in the foot and usually involves both legs. It frequently covers all areas of the foot and leg in a "stocking-glove distribution."

This contrasts with back nerve-related problems or isolated neural problems which are localized and usually involve only one nerve or area of the foot. The loss of sensation response is serious because it can lead to unrecognized injury. Ulcers, infection, and a "Charcot" joint dislocation can follow as a result. See the cases that follow.

Charcot Arthropathy

This severe problem appears to be an extension of diabetic peripheral neuropathy. The Charcot condition can occur any time during the course of diabetes, although its incidence is higher in patients over age forty. Many people with Charcot will have had diabetes for twelve or more years, but some will suffer from it early in the onset of the disease. There is no relationship between the severity of diabetes and Charcot.

The Charcot syndrome is characteristically noticed when there is an onset of severe swelling after a minor ankle sprain or injury. Sometimes it starts with no trauma at all or can appear after more severe injuries such as fractures. The patient's foot is swollen, hot, and red (erythemenous). One can easily mistake it for an infection. Charcot is not an infection, but an early breakdown of the ligaments and tendons leading to severe deformity and joint dislocations. Increased blood supply is usually associated with Charcot. Multiple foot bones begin to dissolve, crumble, and break. Even when the swelling and redness is severe, the patient may have little or no pain. The pain is almost always far less than would be expected by looking at the leg-foot appearance.

A serious aspect of Charcot arthropathy is that it can rapidly develop into a severe deformity, causing pressure ulcers, secondary infections, and eventual amputation. It is the *major reason for amputation* in diabetics when it is not recognized early and aggressively treated. Charcot is a frustrating and difficult problem to care for and treat.

B ill, a forty-year-old government worker, had been diagnosed ten years previously as having diabetes mellitus. His diabetic blood sugars had been hard to control, but with careful monitoring, it has stabilized. He was referred to me by his medical doctor with an "infected" ulcer on the outside of his foot. He said his whole foot and lower leg were in great pain. His pain increased markedly after walking only one block and it was quickly relieved when he rested (claudication). He revealed that he had been a heavy smoker for over fifteen years. Several family members were also diabetics.

His examination showed a quarter-size ulcer on the outside of his small toe (fifth metatarsal) on his right foot. It was NOT on a normal weight-bearing area. His right foot appeared dry, pale, and slightly cool when compared with his left and displayed no normal hair pattern. He was wearing rather narrow pointed toe shoes which were causing pressure on his feet. His x-rays showed no fractures and sensation testing showed a slight decrease in sensitivity. There was only minimal neuropathy. I suspected that his foot ulcer was a secondary symptom of poor blood supply to his foot and sent him for an arteriogram of both legs.

The results showed a significant blockage of blood flow in one of the major thigh arteries as well as blockage in two blood vessels in the calf. His other leg had some blockage as well, but was asymptomatic at that point. Treatment included attempting to heal the ulcer with whirlpool baths, wearing a Darco shoe, and using crutches. The ulcer did not heal and Bill needed a vascular surgeon to reconstruct his leg arteries using bypass grafts. At the same time, he underwent a surgical debridgment on his foot ulcer with removal of a bony prominence that had placed pressure on the area. It was not an infected ulcer but was really a vascular ulcer.

Bill was counseled to stop smoking immediately or the benefits of surgery would be lost. With help, he was able to break the habit and became quite attentive to his diabetes. The ulcer healed over the next six weeks and Bill was able to resume activity without pain. He was careful to wear extra depth shoes. He is followed closely for vascular problems and is a candidate for reconstruction of his left leg arteries.

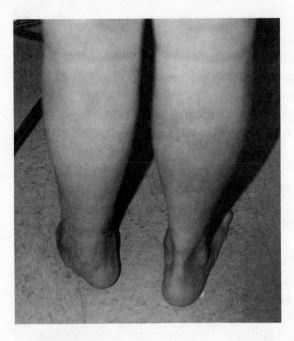

FIGURE 10-2. *Standing Charcot foot deformity (left foot)*

Major Phases

Charcot has three major phases:

1. First is the *bony fragmentation,* ligament disruption phase. Swelling and redness are most severe. Deformity occurs fast and swelling can fluctuate dramatically. The tissue destruction period usually lasts three to six months, but may go on for a year or two. Multiple bones are weakened and tend to break apart.

2. Phase two is the *coalescence phase,* or the stage of repair. The bones tend to harden and joints stiffen (fuse). Swelling, redness, and warmth lessen. These symptoms do not fluctuate like the first stage, which is less stable than phase two. When this second phase is over, there should be no further destruction of the foot or ankle. Unfortunately, forty percent of patients develop Charcot in the other foot or ankle which compounds the problem.

3. In the third phase, there is no significant swelling or redness and the bones are stable. It may take ten months to two years to get to this stage. Unfortunately, the bony deformity is now permanent and may cause more pressure ulcers.

G. H., a forty-five-year-old librarian, was referred to me by the hospital emergency room physician. She had an infected area on her right foot caused by a broken-off needle. She had no memory of stepping on it and went for treatment when her foot became red, swollen, and mildly painful. She was an adult onset diabetic who required insulin injections daily. Her exam showed a loss of muscle contours on her foot, indicating muscle atrophy. There was a marked decrease of sensation in both feet.

In sensation testing, she could not even feel a pinprick on the bottom of her foot. X-rays confirmed that the needle was still in her foot, but there were no fractures or signs of bone infection. Note that soft tissue infections are not seen on regular x-rays.

I surgically drained her infection and removed the needle. She took a two-week course of antibiotics and the wound healed. Swelling persisted, however, and over the next month or two, she developed multiple fractures of the metatarsals, dislocated several small foot joints, and her right foot became quite deformed. She was diagnosed with Charcot neuropathy and was treated with protective casting and crutches for four months until the swelling subsided to prevent further deformity. She was fitted with custom-molded orthotics and special shoes.

Unfortunately, her problems continued. Her left foot began to swell for no apparent reason; no ulcers, bony deformities, or infection were present. The index of suspicion pointed to developing Charcot on her left foot. A special molded cast was applied. However, even with careful casting techniques, this deformity progressed. She developed non-healing ulcers on the bottom of her foot and on the outside of her ankle. She wore the casts until swelling stabilized and the multiple fractures appeared to be healing (stage 3 Charcot). Bracing and special shoes couldn't accommodate the deformity and ulcers recurred. She had surgical straightening, realignment, and fusion (arthrodesis) of her left foot to change pressures back to normal areas and place her foot flat on the floor.

So far, G.H. is functioning well, although the worry is always present that the fusion won't totally heal and secondary infections might occur. Understandably, Charcot surgery has a high incidence of surgical complications because of the nature of this disease.

Ulcers and Infection

There are other major problems associated with Charcot. Pressure ulcers and infection are found in diabetics who have neuropathy with loss of the protective sensation and some skin fissures (breaks in skin). The bony deformity in Charcot causes breaking of the overlying skin. Secondary infections are common, especially in patients with poor blood supply. The diabetic immune system with its lowered white blood cell count does not work well, which promotes infection. Infection is usually in the soft tissues, but may also involve the bone (**osteomyelitis**). It may appear as swelling and redness and is very difficult to differentiate from Charcot. A trained medical professional with extensive experience can properly diagnose these diabetic problems but frequently with considerable difficulty.

A general guideline is to determine if an ulcer which is draining exists in the plantar pad. If so, it is probably infected. Even with infection, however, a patient's temperature may not be elevated. Redness and swelling in the midfoot without an ulcer present is usually a Charcot foot. Many Charcot feet are mistakenly diagnosed as infection and the proper brace or cast for protection is not used. As a result, severe deformity of the foot follows.

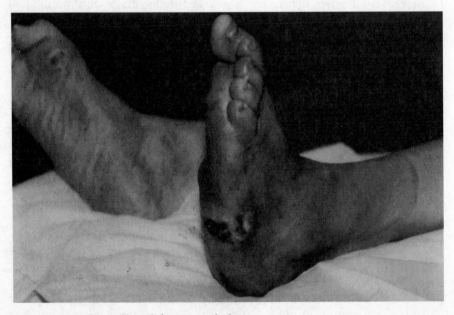

FIGURE 10-3. *Charcot foot deformity and ulcers*

Shirley, a fifty-three-year-old diabetic, was referred to me by her friend. She had experienced persistently red and swollen foot and ankle for four months. Her symptoms developed for no apparent reasons and her medical doctor had treated her for a foot infection by an eight-week course of antibiotics. Her swelling continued and a review of sequential x-rays showed a breaking down of her foot bones. Her doctor diagnosed her condition as osteomyelitis (bone infection) and recommended surgery to remove the infection. He implied that amputation was a strong possibility.

My examination of her foot showed a swollen, mildly red (erythemenous) foot with no ulcers present. Her blood count was close to normal and she had a normal temperature. X-rays showed a mid-foot deformity with multiple bony fractures in this area. The radiologist interpreted this as Charcot arthropathy or osteomyelitis.

My experience with Charcot problems strongly suggested this diagnosis. A needle aspiration was performed to check for pus and deep infection. The results were normal. I sent Shirley for a special bone scan to confirm the Charcot diagnosis. Treatment included special casting for five months until her foot had stabilized. She was then fitted with a brace and special shoe. Her foot does not have a normal appearance, but it rests flat on the floor, and there are no abnormal pressure areas. So far, she is doing well.

It easy to mistake Charcot feet for bone infections. In this case, treatment with antibiotics won't work. It is important to use protective casting to try to decrease the level of deformity.

Self-Help Treatment

From the onset of diabetes, patients must constantly be reminded of potential damage and the need for proper care of their feet. The first principle of therapy and self-help is *patient education* and a *teamwork approach*. There are all kinds of pamphlets and books available about the personal care and prevention of diabetic foot problems. Self-help groups and the Diabetic Foundation are also useful sources for patient and family support. See Appendix C for a list of these sources of support. Poor self-care and lack of treatment are the primary causes leading to amputation.

Here is a critical list for diabetic patients and family members to consider for proper diabetic foot care:

- Do not smoke or drink coffee. Smoking decreases your vascular ability significantly. Nicotine and caffeine also impair circulation. In England and other countries, many vascular surgeons will NOT perform surgical reconstruction if the patient is a smoker.

- Lose weight if you are overweight. Weight adversely affects your blood pressure and hinders your ability to do effective exercises, among other problems. Losing weight is also aesthetically good for mental health and self-esteem.

- Inspect your feet at least once daily and more often if neuropathy is present. Look for blisters, cuts, and redness.

- Inspect between your toes for blisters, cuts, and scratches. If you have poor eyesight, use mirrors, magnifying glasses, or have a family member or a friend provide assistance. See your doctor if any problems occur.

- When comparing your feet, check if one feels warmer than the other.

- Avoid extremes in temperature. Before getting into the tub, check the water temperature to make sure it is not too hot.

- Wash your feet daily and dry them carefully, especially between your toes. Use only powder between your toes. Use lotion on the rest of your foot.

- For dry skin, use a light coat of baby oil and then wipe dry with a towel.

- Do *not* use chemicals, especially corn or callus remover on your feet.

- Do *not* walk barefoot, as the diabetic foot can be less sensitive to objects in general.

- Inspect the insides of your shoes and shake them out daily—more often if you have neuropathy. Also, do not wear shoes without stockings.

- Do not wear constricting socks, socks with seams, mended socks, or garters. Wear natural fibers, preferably cotton, as they tend to absorb moisture. Dry feet are less susceptible to inflammation or infection.

- Have your health care provider's phone number available and be sure there is coverage during nonworking hours.

- Do not walk on hot surfaces like pool decks or sandy beaches.

- Do not use adhesive tape on your feet.

- Avoid trimming your corns or calluses. Use a pumice stone gently after washing if it is absolutely necessary.

- Trim your nails only straight across at the level of the tips of the toes and no shorter. If you have eyesight or flexibility problems, have a trained specialist do it. Realistically speaking, you should seek expert assistance in trimming your toenails. Accidental cuts can lead to serious infections. "Bathroom surgery" (patients conveniently trimming their toenails, corns, and so on before or after taking a bath) of any kind is strictly forbidden.

- Do not wear tight, ill-fitting shoes that can irritate your feet or cause inflammation and swelling. Proper shoes are essential. Extra depth, soft soles with inserts, or loose or velcro closings are recommended. Check your new shoes with care for comfort and proper fit. See chapter 15 on shoe fitting.

- Ensure that your doctor or health care provider inspects your feet at each visit. If you have a neuropathy, your feet should be examined at least once every two or three months.

- Exercise is the best therapy available to the patient. It helps control appetite in diabetic persons who need to lose weight. Diabetics who exercise regularly are also better able to control their condition than those who don't. Exercise your feet up and down or walk regularly. Pump your feet to improve circulation. A brisk walk should suffice for those unable to do more strenuous exercises.

- Elevate your feet when you are sitting and avoid crossing your legs as it constricts blood vessels.

- Before you get into a tub, check the water temperature to make sure it is not too hot. If you have reduced nerve function, you may have difficulty judging temperature. Remember that scalded feet do not heal quickly.

Medical Treatment

There are several *warning red flags* for diabetic foot patients. In each case, see your doctor right away!

- Minor infections—there are NO minor infections among diabetics.

- Infected toenails—frequently progress to main infection. They are among the most common nail problems and can lead to disastrous infection, even amputation, if cut improperly.

- Swelling—may indicate Charcot.

- Injury—sprained ankle and fractures must be treated longer in diabetic patients. Frequently, they turn into or reveal the presence of a Charcot problem. Casting is often required.

Swelling, redness, or infection in a diabetic patient is a medical EMERGENCY. Your medical doctor needs to be familiar with all aspects of diabetes and be readily available. Routine eye checks, kidney, and vascular exams should be done regularly. Good control of your blood sugar is also essential. Proper diet management is very important and you may need the help of a nutritionist to ensure the right balance.

To ensure proper diagnosis of infection versus Charcot arthropathy, it is recommended that you see an appropriate infectious disease specialist and a foot specialist. Appropriate x-rays are needed and a bone scan (indium) may help in diagnosis. In this test, dye is injected into a vein and will accumulate in the area of the bone problem.

For an acute soft tissue infection or abscess, an MRI (magnetic resonance imaging) may be needed. Unfortunately, MRI does not distinguish foot infection from Charcot. Finally, a biopsy or aspiration may be prescribed. This invasive procedure should be done only after meticulous cleaning of the involved area. The problem with this approach is the risk of infection.

If the diabetic patient develops a foot ulcer, the cause must be identified. If it is caused by vascular blockage, areas of pale skin, decreased hair growth, and abnormal pulses need to be evaluated. You might have to see a vascular surgeon who may perform an ultrasound test or an arteriogram. In this test, dye is injected into a leg artery to give a picture of the vessels. Toe blood pressure Doppler tests (ultrasound way to examine blood flow in an artery), NOT ankle blood pressure measurement, is an excellent screening tool to identify vascular disease.

If the ulcer is caused by bony pressure, the deformity must be properly padded and proper shoes or inserts/orthotics are necessary. A shoe/support specialist is frequently consulted for assistance. Special casting (total contact casts) may be needed to distribute pressures on the foot more evenly and control swelling. If infection is present, appropriate cultures must be taken to identify the bacteria. Antibiotic treatment is then initiated.

We should emphasize the importance of correctly identifying the Charcot foot. During the first destructive phase, medical treatment includes total contact casting or bracing to prevent further foot deformity and control swelling. Wrapping and other treatments are sometimes used, but are not as successful and do not prevent subsequent severe foot deformity. The first six weeks of casting are non-weight bearing. This is followed by a prolonged period of weight bearing casts for three to nine months or longer. The cast must be changed frequently at first (as it loosens), because swelling decreases. Once swelling has stabilized, the cast does not need to be changed as frequently and even bracing may be effective. Some patients require a permanent brace or a custom shoe.

Remember that routine foot or ankle injuries and fractures must be treated with protection for a much longer period in diabetic patients. These injuries may trigger Charcot.

Surgical Treatment

Complications relating to diabetes often require surgery. But for diabetic sufferers, surgery has complications of its own. Diabetes itself hampers the body's ability to heal surgical wounds. The diabetic with severe vascular disease can benefit from much improved surgical techniques to reconstruct blood flow to the foot. It may need to be combined with foot ulcer surgery before the foot ulcer will heal. There are no surgical techniques to restore better nerve function in the foot. But when a deformity occurs or pressure problems develop as secondary symptoms to the neuropathy, surgical procedures may be necessary to correct these deformities.

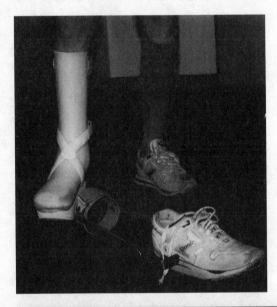

Before considering surgery, try corrected shoes, inserts, or braces. For severe Charcot foot deformities that cannot be helped this way, surgery may be needed. It is rarely done until the bone is in the healing phase. Usually, the deformed bump is removed. When severe deformity exists, bone fusion and stabilization using plates, screws, rods,

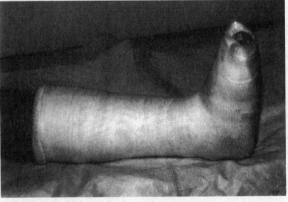

FIGURE 10-4. *Total contact cast (left) and AFO brace with Rocker sole shoe and brace (above)*

staples, and other devices are used for fixation. This is one reason why an orthopedic surgeon is sometimes called the carpenter of surgery. A prolonged period of casting is required after the procedure, lasting from six to nine months. Sometimes electrical stimulation is applied (bone stimulator) to assist the healing process.

For simpler toe deformities, hammertoe procedures may be done. When the metatarsal head is applying pressure, it may need to be removed surgically. Unfortunately, this sometimes transfers stress to other areas of the foot.

Surgical treatment of infection is occasionally recommended. It includes draining the infection, leaving the wound open to properly drain, or debridement and removal of the infected bone. Once bone infection (osteomyelitis) has occurred, eradication of this problem is very difficult.

Expectations and Complications

The diabetic foot patient should consider being at risk for foot problems throughout life. Some vascular reconstruction is successful, but the small vessels of the foot are not likely to be salvageable. Amputation of part of the foot or leg (rarely above the knee) may have to be done. The same holds for the severely deformed Charcot foot. There is a high rate of infection. Failure of the bone to fuse and further collapse may also occur after Charcot surgery. If a proper weight bearing foot cannot be assured, ulcers and infection that occur may lead to amputation.

Today's amputation techniques are much improved, as lighter and more manageable materials are now available. There are also special foot amputations that attempt to avoid higher amputations of the limb. They are quite successful, helping the patient regain functionality. Determining the correct level of amputation is exacting and requires both careful evaluation and an experienced skillful surgeon.

It should be stressed that amputation is no easy decision. In addition to medical and physical factors, the patient's mental state and readiness to accept the fact that losing one or both feet means a change in activities and lifestyle are important for rehabilitation. Although in many cases, there is no choice but to amputate, preparing the patient for the impending loss of his or her natural "transportation system" is a critical first step. Support groups are available. See Appendix C.

Treating infection with antibiotics has a downside. The antibiotics required are often quite powerful and may damage the kidney or liver, or cause cross-reactions if other medicines are being taken. Prolonged use of antibiotics may lead to secondary growth of more resistant infectious organisms. This is where an infectious disease specialist should be called to assist in managing and monitoring infection in the diabetic patient.

IN A NUTSHELL

Diabetes is a serious disease that can have a disastrous effect on your feet. It is very important for you to know a lot about this disease and to work closely with your doctor to control symptoms. You need to take good care of your feet and examine them every day. If you find any unusual redness, swelling, or sores, see your doctor IMMEDIATELY. Diabetes complications like Charcot or ulcers are serious and develop quickly. Family members and diabetic patients need to take responsibility to help in proper diabetic foot care.

DOCTOR'S CORNER: QUESTIONS AND ANSWERS

In the past, I have had diabetic foot problems but I'm not having trouble with my feet now. Why does my doctor want to see me every few months?

It is important to have your feet inspected carefully each time you go to your medical doctor. You should also get assistance in trimming your nails as cuts can lead to infection. If your doctor finds any neuropathy, it needs to be evaluated at least every two to three months to monitor any progressing foot deformity or problems. Diabetic foot problems can progress quickly.

My blood sugar is pretty well controlled. Why do I still have so much trouble with skin ulcers on my feet?

Your skin ulcers suggest that you might have peripheral neuropathy with some associated foot deformity that causes pressure on certain areas of your feet. It is also possible that you have a vascular (circulation) problem that causes these ulcers. Blood sugar control is very important, but unfortunately some problems can still occur from diabetes.

I twisted my ankle slightly yesterday and today it is very swollen. What should I do?

Whenever swelling occurs in diabetic patients, seek help immediately. Swelling is considered an emergency. It could just be a symptom of a minor injury, but it could also be a forewarning of Charcot arthropathy or infection with disastrous implications. GET MEDICAL ATTENTION FAST.

TERMS TO REMEMBER

Arteriogram: Dye injected into a leg artery to show a picture of the arteries in order to determine the circulation and/or areas of blockage.

Atrophy: Loss of normal muscle size, appearance, and function.

Charcot: Degenerative disorder of the central and peripheral nervous system of the foot; an early breakdown of ligaments and tendons leading to deformities and joint dislocations.

Charcot arthropathy: A progressive bone, ligament, and tendon–destructive disease that is related to neuropathy. It can result in severe foot deformity.

Claudication: See intermittent claudication.

Debridement: The surgical removal of infected or dead tissue and foreign matter.

Diabetes: A system disease or disorder caused by the body's inability to transport sugar from blood to cells, causing vessels to harden and reducing blood flow to the arteries.

Diabetes mellitus: The medical term for diabetes.

Gangrene: Death of the tissue from lack of blood supply.

Hyperglycemia: Blood sugar that is too low or too high.

Intermittent claudication: A condition caused by circulation problems that creates pain and cramps in the legs during exercise and is relieved during rest.

Ischemia: Vascular deficiency (lack of circulation) from a blockage of arterial blood flow that results in poor oxygen supply and death of tissue, unless circulation is restored.

Neuropathy: When the nerve supply is diseased. The diseased nerve may cause sensation (feeling) abnormalities, loss of muscle function, or autosurvic nerve malfunction (poor, sweaty), or all of these.

Osteomyelitis: Bone infection. It is a serious problem and hard to eradicate.

Peripheral neuropathy: When the nerve supply to muscle is diseased, the muscle does not function and becomes atrophied. Some muscles function better than their opposite partners, causing muscle imbalance.

Ulcer: A break in the continuity of tissue; an open sore which often leads to a total breakdown of the underlying tissue and becomes infected.

CHAPTER 11

Arthritis—What Does It Mean to Me?

*I am interested in physical medicine
Because my father was. I am interested
in medical research because I believe in it.
I am interested in arthritis, because I have it.*

—BERNARD M. BARUCH

Arthritis is wear and tear in a body joint which comes with age and can be an inherited disease. The fact that it is treatable means early diagnosis and regular prescribed exercises to ensure a satisfactory lifestyle. Surgery is the last resort, depending on the stage of the disease and cause of the symptoms.

INTRODUCTION

The word arthritis comes from two Greek words: *Arthra* which means joint and *itis* meaning inflammation or swelling. *Arthritis* is a general term for swelling of the lining and cartilage damage of joints. It is a "wearing out" of the shock absorbing ends of the bone (cartilage) at the surface of the joint like the hip joint, knee joint, or one of the foot joints.

Cartilage is a soft tissue that acts as a buffer between bone ends. When arthritis sets in, this soft tissue weakens, exposing the bone and allowing thick fluid to reside in the joint. The cells that hold fluid as lubricant begin to secrete too much fluid which swells the joints—an early sign of joint inflammation and an indicator that something is wrong within the joint.

As you can deduce, arthritis is not a disease but a wear-and-tear process in a body joint that precipitates an inflammation due to a breakdown in the cartilage tissue. Would you expect the best tires on your car to last forever? Excessive biomechanical forces (pressures on the joints) contribute to this condition, so overweight individuals subject their joints to more wear and tear than others, even with less strenuous activities.

When a biomechanical malalignment is present, more excessive wear and tear takes place in your limbs. Knock kneed and bowlegged adults are illustrations of how poor biomechanics of the foot throw out the alignment of your body and cause excessive stress on certain joints from the lower back down.

"I have arthritis, doctor, and sooner or later I'm scared that I'll be in a wheelchair and crippled" is a statement I hear from some of my patients. The first job is to reassure these frightened people that most arthritis problems can be treated, the symptoms of this disease can usually be controlled, and the quality of life can be good—even with severe arthritis.

NATURAL HISTORY

There are various causes of arthritis; the symptoms, progression, and possible disability depend on the type of arthritis you have. There are more than 100 forms of arthritis affecting over 37 million Americans.

The most common are:

- Osteoarthritis (degenerative arthritis)
- Rheumatoid arthritis and its variants
- Systemic lupus erythematosis
- Gouty arthritis
- Psoriasis

WHAT'S IN A JOINT?

Before we talk about arthritis and its many ramifications, we should expose you to the basic anatomy of the joint. The various parts of a joint are:

- **Articular cartilage**—shock absorbing elastic tissue covering the ends of bone.
- **Synovium**—the lining of the joint which produces synovial fluid.
- **Synovial fluid**—the lubricating fluid of joints. Excess synovial fluid is produced when inflammation is present.
- **Joint capsule**—the supportive tissue holding the two joint bones together.
- **Ligaments**—additional supportive structures just outside the joint which provide stability.
- **Subchondral bone**—the hard bone just beneath the cartilage that provides support for the cartilage. See figure 11-1.

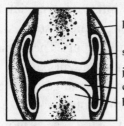

knee ligament

synovium (joint lining)

joint fluid (synovial fluid)
cartilage (covers end of bone)
bone (underneath cartilage)

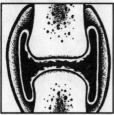
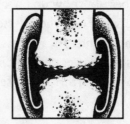

FIGURE 11-1. *Normal joint (above), mild arthritic joint (below left), and severe ankle arthritic joint (below right).*

OSTEOARTHRITIS—A DEGENERATIVE JOINT DISEASE OR MECHANICAL ARTHRITIS

Natural History

Osteoarthritis is the most common type of arthritis. It has been estimated to affect about 90 percent of people over age sixty. Sixteen million Americans have been diagnosed with this disease. It is associated with aging, affecting primarily the weight bearing joints (back, hips, knees, and feet). This joint abnormality may affect one or more joints.

The cause of osteoarthritis is unknown and no one seems to understand why some people develop this type more acutely than others. For example, people whose x-rays show the same degree of joint degeneration may experience different symptoms: one experiences intense pain while another no symptoms at all.

Traumatic arthritis, which occurs when a fracture of one of the joint bones takes place, is identical to osteoarthritis. Microscopic examination and x-rays show the same disease. This implies that minor or sometimes major trauma plays a role in arthritis development. Arthritis starts when the cartilage cells that maintain the joint cartilage break down. During the early stages, the cartilage covering the end of the bone breaks off into the joint. This causes a secondary inflammation of the joint lining (synovium) which reacts by producing excessive inflamed synovial fluid. Associated swelling can also cause a feeling of tightness, stiffness, and pain by stretching the pain nerves located in the lining. There may be mild, severe, continuous, or, more commonly, intermittent pain.

In the early stages of traumatic arthritis, very few changes are seen on x-rays. Since cartilage is the same density as other soft tissues like ligaments and tendons, it does not show up on x-rays. However, as more and more layers of cartilage wear out, the affected joint space becomes narrowed compared to other joints. As arthritis worsens, the bone ends get bigger and even form spurs (osteophytes). These joint spurs are unique to osteoarthritis or traumatic arthritis and separates them from rheuma-

B ill, an avid thirty-eight-year-old avoid motorcycle rider, was thrown from his motorcycle at high speed. He fractured and dislocated his left ankle. I reduced his ankle (put it back in place) in the emergency room, but did not feel that the reduction was acceptable. Joint injuries need to be put back together in as close a position to the original anatomy as possible. I performed surgery on the patient and his bones were relocated into a better position by using a plate and screws.

Even with good surgical reduction, the severity of this injury can often cause arthritis. Bill continued to have progressive pain in his ankle. It had swelling and loss of motion. Over the next several months, he was treated with common arthritis treatments of NSAIDs, moist heat, and physical therapy for range of motion. Sequential x-rays of Bill's ankle showed a loss of joint space (the cartilage covering bone).

Many people can live quite satisfactorily with arthritis, but Bill's quality of life was disrupted by his limitations and pain. He elected to have additional surgery to fuse his ankle. He was in a series of casts for three months. The ankle fused but swelling persisted. He wore compression stockings and a special shoe with a cushioned heel and a rocker sole to relieve ankle stress. His rehabilitation time was prolonged, but within a year, he functioned very well and has no noticeable limp. He is very happy to have his life back.

toid arthritis. The spurs are *not* painful, but are part of the body's reaction to the arthritis process. Eventually, most of the bony end surface cartilage will be eroded and bone begins rubbing against bone (creaking). When this happens, leg or foot deformity begins and pain becomes more severe and disabling.

It should be noted that there are no pain nerves in cartilage. So even though early arthritis indicates a worn joint, until the underlying bone with its pain nerve fibers is exposed, there will be only mild aching, stiffness, or discomfort. The patient's activity level gradually becomes more and more restricted.

The most common areas affected by osteoarthritis:

1. Low back

2. Neck

3. Hips

4. Knees

5. Ankle—hindfoot

6. Great toe—MTP joint

7. Metatarsal—midtarsal joints (lisfranc)

8. Fingers (herberdens nodes)—enlarged knobs at the end (DISTAL) or middle finger joints

Fortunately, in most osteoarthritis sufferers, the symptoms of the disease remain mild throughout their lifetime. Progression is usually very slow. But once osteoarthritis is diagnosed, the rapidity of destruction and the worsening of symptoms are not predictable. Rest assured that, unlike other forms of arthritis, osteoarthritis is not associated specifically with other medical problems.

RHEUMATOID ARTHRITIS

The next most common arthritis is rheumatoid arthritis which affects about one in five arthritis victims. There are over 2.5 million Americans afflicted with this abnormality. Rheumatoid arthritis begins in the soft tissue surrounding the joint. Early in the course of this disease, the joint lining (synovium) and lining around tendons become inflamed. This produces fluid, warmth, and swelling within and around the joint. The natural history after this point is quite variable.

Rheumatoid arthritis can start at any age and involves one of multiple joints including joints in the arms, back, or legs. There seems to be a genetic predisposition and women are at risk three times more than men.

This may be related to an immune deficiency or possibly a virus or infectious cause. Thirty-five percent of the people experience only *one* attack without recurrent problems or significant arthritis. Between 2 and 3 percent of our population (average age fifty-five) will develop this disease. One half of those with the disease experience recurrent attacks. Eventually, their joints malfunction and become severely arthritic. Only 15 percent of rheumatoid arthritis sufferers experience progressive *continuous* disease and deformity. See figure 11-2.

It is important to remember that rheumatoid arthritis has many levels of severity. The inflammation begins with no apparent cause in the joint lining. As the soft tissue inflammation continues, the tendons become degenerated and torn and the joint capsules destroyed. This leads to muscle imbalance, joint dislocations, and associated deformities. Erosion and the wearing out of the joint is followed by the ultimate development of permanent arthritis. Many other systems may be involved to include the lungs, vascular system, and so on. The feet are affected as well. The first victims are the toes or forefoot (MTP) joints, followed by the hindfoot (subtaler and midtarsal joints). Ankle arthritis may occur, but is less common.

Common Foot Deformities from Rheumatoid Arthritis

There are several foot deformities that are triggered by rheumatoid arthritis:

- Bunions
- Flat feet (50 percent)
- Claw toes
- Metatarsalgia and calluses
- Swollen ankles
- Nodules
- Morton's neuroma.

TREATMENT FOR FOOT ARTHRITIS

This treatment is for all types of foot arthritis, unless it is otherwise specified.

Self-Help Treatment

Though rheumatoid arthritis is a serious illness, experts agree that with appropriate treatment most sufferers improve substantially and experience fewer symptoms. All foot arthritis can be helped by shock absorption and shoes to fit the patient's deformity (extra depth, soft soles). Shoes do not correct deformities, but help reduce pain and pressure. See figure 11-3.

Over-the-counter shoe inserts or arch supports, like Spenko or Sorbuthane may also provide comfort. A shoe with a wider and deeper toe box is important for arthritis sufferers. If your job or activities require standing on hard surfaces like marble or concrete, placing a cushioned mat or rug on the floor will alleviate generalized aching in the foot and legs.

Moist heat, warm soaks, and hot tub baths should relax the joints at least temporarily. Using ice after activities helps alleviate swelling (inflammation) and pain. Aspirin or NSAIDs are commonly used to relieve general aches, pains, and inflammation.

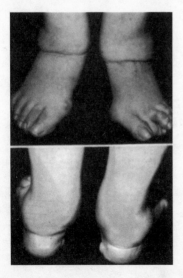

Gentle exercise helps maintain joint mobility and relieve painful symptoms. The type of exercise and equipment used (treadmills, bikes, and so on) vary from individual to individual. Try not to overstress joints. Lose weight if you are overweight. A one pound loss relieves three pounds of pressure on the hip joint. You may also have to alter your life style by

FIGURE 11-2. *Rheumatoid arthritis*

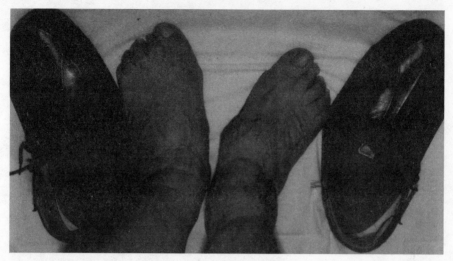

FIGURE 11-3. *Rheumatoid arthritic feet and shoes*

weight. A one pound loss relieves three pounds of pressure on the hip joint. You may also have to alter your life style by selecting activities that accommodate your arthritis. The senior author has given up tennis, but now finds that he enjoys golf as much or more.

Medical Treatment

The cause of your arthritis should be determined by your medical doctor or even an arthritis specialist—a rheumatologist. He or she will perform specific blood tests, take x-rays, and other tests to evaluate your arthritis. NSAIDs may be tried for a short course or, in some cases, a prolonged one. The treatment should be monitored to make sure no side problems are caused by these drugs. The rheumatologist may use other drugs for resistant cases of arthritis. The problem won't cure the disease, but may relieve symptoms and alter the inflammation process. Some of the drugs used are:

- Methotrexate
- Gold
- D-penicillinamine
- Anti-malarial medicines
- Steroids

Injections of cortisone (steroids) into the joint may be used for severely symptomatic and medically resistant arthritis. Physical therapy is often prescribed for specific modalities and exercises. They include:

- Cold therapy for acute pain.
- Moist heat (104 degrees) for lingering pain.
- Contrast—cold followed by heat. You should avoid heat if you have vasculities and avoid cold if you have Raynads phenomena (extreme sensitivity to cold).
- Ultrasound (deep heat).
- Exercises and stretching.
- Gentle motion exercises for the ankle and toes to maintain motion.
- Custom shoes or accommodative shoes (similar to diabetic shoes) may be required.

Occasionally, leg braces like the AFO (ankle foot orthosis) or metal upright braces are prescribed. The purpose of these devices is to limit painful arthritis motion or hold the leg/foot in a more proper alignment.

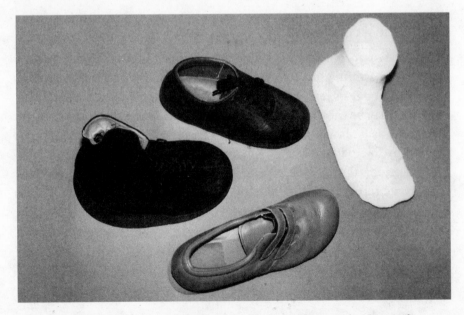

FIGURE 11-4. *Custom and extra depth shoes (laces or velcro) and cotton sock*

Surgical Treatment

If self-help and medical treatments are unsuccessful, surgery becomes an option. Performing surgery and the procedure to follow depend on the stage of the disease and the cause of the troublesome symptoms. For example, pressure symptoms from dysfunctional joints caused by soft tissue imbalances are corrected by tendon releases. If an abnormal angle of the bones is the culprit, then osteotomy (bone realignment) of the toes or hindfoot may be necessary. See chapter 5.

Rheumatoid arthritis is primarily due to the destruction caused by the synovium. So bone realignments (osteotomies) to straighten toes or the hindfoot and save the joints rarely work. Predictably, the joints will become more arthritic and deformed. If the pain symptoms are severe enough or the deformity is great enough to cause abnormal stress on other joints (especially the knees), a stabilization procedure (fusion) should be considered. Unfortunately, to date there are no successful long-lasting artificial joints for the hindfoot or ankle. Some new toe joint replacements are being tried, but their long-term success rates are still in question.

The commonly fused joints for arthritis are the following:

1. Triple arthrodesis (midtarsal and subtaler joints). Frequently performed to relieve painful deformed flat foot problems or other hindfoot deformities.

2. Ankle joint. Arthrodesis is the only reliable procedure for treating a painful ankle for a patient with rheumatoid arthritis.

3. Great toe (MTP) joint. It is a good procedure for arthritis and severe bunion problems of the great toe.

4. Distal joint of the toe for hammertoe or mallet toe problems.

5. Lisfranc (metatarsal—tarsal). This procedure is occasionally done for osteoarthritis, but less so for rheumatoid arthritis.

In rheumatoid arthritis patients, if the joint lining remains persistently swollen, painful, and resistant to medical treatment, the recommended approach is removal of that joint's or that tendon's lining (synovectomy). This is usually done before significant arthritis has become established. In most cases, it seems to slow the progression of the disease and/or at least significantly relieve pain symptoms.

There are two commonly performed soft tissue procedures:

1. Synovectomy of the MTP joints of the toes—diagnosed by pain and swelling in the ball of the foot.

2. Synovectomy of the lining of tendons—an attempt to prevent tendon rupture when medical treatment has not worked.

In rheumatoid patients with claw toes, metatarsalgia, and severe arthritis, we use the Hoffman procedure which requires removal of the ends of the metatarsals ("the marbles").

Expectations and Complications of Treatment

Whether medical or surgical, the treatment is not always successful and complications can occur. The possible risks versus the potential gains of any treatment must be carefully evaluated by the patient and physician:

- Stomach problems or stomach ulcers affect two percent of people taking NSAIDs or aspirin. On rare occasions, liver or kidney function can be disturbed. That is the primary reason why careful monitoring is highly recommended. It is especially important to monitor bowel movements for a black appearance or fresh blood. DO NOT continue taking the medicine if any symptoms occur.

- Rheumatoid arthritis drugs are powerful and require medical management. For example, cortisone (prednisone and other steroids) have a number of side effects. Over time, they may be hard to control and must be considered when surgery is planned. Methatrexate is discontinued before surgery because it appears to alter wound healing.

- Repeated injections into joints tend to weaken cartilage, tendons, and ligaments and should be used only after carefully weighing the risk versus the gain.

- Habit forming pain medicines should be used cautiously and infrequently.

- Surgery is often successful in relieving specific joint pain, but may transfer stress to other joints causing further deformity. The surgical decision needs to be based on specific goals to relieve deformity —hopefully, preventing destruction of other joints and relieving pain. As can be seen from the case below, no surgery is guaranteed. You should have a careful understanding of goals, expectations (long-term benefits), and complications. See chapter 17.

P am, a petite thirty-five-year-old with severe rheumatoid arthritis in multiple joints, was referred to me by her orthopedic surgeon. He had performed bilateral total knee replacements to straighten her knock-knees and relieve her pain. Now she was having trouble with her feet. Pam noticed they were getting flatter and becoming very painful.

X-rays showed a progressive loss of her foot joint spaces and dislocations of the small joints. Her right foot deformity had become severe and her hind foot joints had become quite displaced. She was walking on the inside bones of her foot and was quite disabled.

She was fitted for special shoes with medial (inside) heel flares and medial extended heel counters to try to hold her foot in a better weight-bearing position. This was not successful, so she elected to have surgery. She had a fusion of her hind foot (triple arthrodesis) to hold her foot straight. She had three months of casting and physical therapy to regain ankle motion.

Her pain was relieved and now she can wear non-custom shoes. Unfortunately, her left foot is progressing in its deformity and will probably require surgery in the near future.

Other Arthritis

The medical treatment for other forms of arthritis is similar to either osteoarthritis or rheumatoid arthritis treatment. Proper diagnosis is important, however, because of associated medical problems and to choose the correct medicine.

Gout

Gout is the painful result of a chemical metabolism problem associated with elevated crystals of uric acid—a chemical produced by the liver that settles in and around various joint tissues; it passes out of the body in the urine. Men suffer from gout eight or nine times more frequently than pre-menopausal women. The disease appears to run in families. The big toes, heels, or knees (a favorite site for arthritis) are commonly affected in most cases of gout probably because they are subject to continued pressure in walking.

The stress of surgery can cause a flareup of gout or even its first occurrence. It is not uncommon to have kidney stones, as well. The gout flareup or the kidney stone experience will be embedded in your memory as one of the most painful experiences—ever!

As you can tell, gout is a chronic disease that normally begins with recurring attacks, followed by periods of remission. Most sufferers experience repeated attacks throughout their lives. When an attack comes, it can last eight to ten days. The joint becomes swollen and painful. The skin above it sometimes turns red or even purple. The use of diuretics or "water pills," or a rapid loss of tissue from crash dieting, can trigger the settling of uric acid in the bloodstream, causing problems.

Your doctor sometimes treats gout with anti-inflammatory drugs that increase uric acid excretion or drugs which reduce uric acid production. Indocin appears to be the most effective NSAID to treat the acute attack. Steroid injection can also be administered to relieve pain, although it does not eliminate the cause. The best advice is to rest during a gout attack and take your body weight off the affected joints. Drink a lot of water to dilute the uric acid salts in the kidneys. Surgery is the last resort—in situations where your joint is badly damaged and in pain. In such a case, remodeling the joint or other types of arthritis joint surgeries may be needed.

Other Diseases

There are other diseases that affect the foot and are similar to rheumatoid arthritis. These are:

- **Ankylosing spondylitis.** This is mainly hip and back arthritis, but resistant heel pain and MTP joint inflammation may occur.

- **Psoriasis.** Often, arthritis occurs before the skin rash appears. The hands, feet, and heel pads are also involved. It may be associated with Reiter's syndrome and Rheumatoid arthritis.

- **Reiter's syndrome.** Eye inflammation (conjunctivitis), genital inflammation or discharge, bowel inflammation, and a nonsymmetrical arthritis (not the same on both feet) or a swollen toe are the symptoms. It appears to be an infectious disease and is self-limited. HIV patients may be associated with Reiter's syndrome or psoriasis. Taking Immunosuppressive medicines may have serious side effects.

- **Lyme disease.** This is a tick infection, that, in its later stages, can involve the foot and ankle. Tendinitis, joint pains, and plantar fasciitis are symptoms. It occurs in endemic areas of the northeast, Minnesota, and California (in 10 regions). It is now covering nine states.

Overall, the index of suspicion is the key to diagnosing and successfully treating arthritis.

IN A NUTSHELL

Most arthritis is osteoarthritis or mechanical arthritis which results in wear and tear of your joints. Remember that most arthritis problems can be treated and the cause of your arthritis should be diagnosed. Simple treatments like warm soaks, ice, NSAIDs, and stretching exercises will help relieve many arthritis symptoms.

Rheumatoid arthritis needs to be treated by an arthritis specialist to relieve severe joint inflammations and to treat deformities in joints that can occur.

DOCTOR'S CORNER: QUESTIONS AND ANSWERS

I have just been diagnosed as having osteoarthritis in my knees. Does this mean that I'll get arthritis in my foot and ankles next?

You won't necessarily get arthritis anywhere else, but if you do get arthritis in your feet or ankles, it will probably be less severe and progressive. There are no successful joint replacements for joints in the foot or ankle, so conservative treatment is the first line of defense.

I have just had my great toe fused because of arthritis. What limitations can I expect now?

Depending on the position of your fixed great toe, the height of the heel you wear is limited. Lower heels are more tolerated than higher heels. You will have no observable limp and with the proper adjustments in your shoes, like a rocker sole, you may find that jogging is possible. The pain you had will be dramatically relieved, so any limits on your activities from pain before surgery will most likely be gone.

I have just been diagnosed with rheumatoid arthritis. Will it affect all of my joints sooner or later?

Rheumatoid arthritis has many presentations and forms in the disease. You may have a few joints or many chronically involved during the course of the disease. It just isn't possible to predict this at the beginning stages of this arthritis. The foot is commonly involved in rheumatoid arthritis and usually responds to proper footwear and cushioning.

I have rheumatoid arthritis and have claw toes with severe pain under the metatarsal pads. I have calluses there, too. What do you suggest?

This is the most common rheumatoid arthritis foot problem and it starts with an inflammation of the synovium (joint lining) of the toe joints. It develops into severe arthritis of the MTP joints and has associated dislocations. This causes the clawing of the toes. When severe calluses and deformities are present and they don't respond to adequate cushioning and appropriate shoes, surgery can be very beneficial. It involves removing the metatarsal heads by the Hoffman procedure. The foot may be slightly shorter, but pain is dramatically relieved and the relief is usually lasting. When both feet are involved, surgery can be performed on them at the same time.

TERMS TO REMEMBER

Ankylosing spondylitis: Mainly hip and back arthritis, but resistant heel pain and MTP joint inflammation may be present.

Articular cartilage: Shock absorbing elastic tissue covering the ends of bone.

Arthritis: A general term for swelling of the lining and cartilage of joints.

Cartilage: A soft tissue that acts as a buffer between bone ends.

Gout: A chronic disease—a painful result of a chemical metabolism problem associated with elevated crystals of uric acid settling in and around various joint tissues.

Hoffman procedure: A surgical procedure that requires the removal of the ends of the metatarsals.

Joint capsule: The supportive tissue holding the two joint bones together.

Ligament: An additional supportive structure just outside the joint which provides stability.

Reiter's syndrome: An infectious disease showing symptoms such as eye inflammation, genital inflammation/discharge, bowel inflammation, or swollen toe.

Subchondral bone: The hard bone just beneath the cartilage that provides support for the cartilage.

Synovectomy: Surgery to remove an inflamed joint lining that often includes the rerouting of tendons.

Synovial fluid: The lubricating fluid of joints. Excess synovial fluid is produced when inflammation is present.

Synovium: The lining of the joint which produces synovial fluid.

Triple arthrodesis: Surgical procedure to fuse and stabilize the midtarsal and subtaler joints to relieve painful flat foot or other hindfoot deformities.

CHAPTER 12

Common Sports Injuries and Fractures of the Foot and Ankle

When I was forty, my doctor advised me that a man in his forties shouldn't play tennis. I heeded his advice carefully and could hardly wait until I reached fifty to start again.

—JUSTICE HUGO BLACK, quoted in *Think*, Feb., 1963

Sports are a useful activity to people of all ages as long as they maintain safe and prudent habits to avoid injuries. A "nothing in excess" attitude is good advice to follow. When experiencing difficulties (fractures, tendinitis, and so on.), follow self-help treatment and consult your doctor accordingly.

INTRODUCTION

For over a decade, we have been witnessing a steady increase in organized and recreational sports for all age groups—men, women, and young adults. The surge of sports and athletics has been accompanied by a significant increase in injuries sustained by these athletes. Most of the injuries are cuts and bruises. Some injuries are more serious, requiring medical attention, hospitalization, and even surgery.

When something hurts, it is nature's way of telling us that we ought to slow down or stop and rest. We also need to find out what is causing the discomfort. The most common complaints are from stress or injuries related to the foot and ankle.

Sports injuries can be caused by acute injury or trauma related directly to the "hazards" of a particular sport. On the other hand, they may be related to overload or repetitive stress. This latter problem often goes untreated or undertreated, prolonging the athlete's recovery time. Even the "simple" ankle sprain (the most common acute soft tissue injury) occurring in sports, is NOT so simple. It needs to be treated as a serious injury because it can lead to prolonged recovery or chronic problems.

In this chapter, we define and discuss chronic stress injuries such as stress fractures, tendinitis, and shin splints. Included are guidelines on how to identify your problem and when to get help. The common acute ankle and foot fractures and sprains are also explained. You need to know what to expect in the way of recovery time and the long-term effects of such problems.

NATURAL HISTORY OF OVER-STRESS INJURIES: STRESS FRACTURES AND TENDINITIS

As mentioned in previous chapters, our bodies continue throughout life to adjust to the various and changing physical life forces by structurally remodeling. Children rapidly adapt their bone, ligament, and tendon structures to changing pressures. Adults adapt as well, but at a slower rate.

Overworking our bodies can lead to stress fracture and tendinitis. Stress fracture is a painful reaction of bone that occurs when the stress applied to it has exceeded the bone's ability to withstand or remodel to that stress. Tendinitis is a painful reaction in a tendon when excess stress has been applied. To illustrate the point, read Tina's case below and see what you think.

This particular case demonstrates the classical history of the *stress reaction syndrome*. The patient has changed rather quickly to a more rigorous activity level. Typically, the overstress will continue for three to four weeks followed by rather abrupt (acute) pain in the overstressed area. This is sometimes associated with mild swelling. If sequential weekly examinations of the bone or tendon were done under a microscope from the beginning of stress to the time symptoms began, dramatic cellular changes would be seen. An increase in blood flow is channeled to the stressed area to allow it to adapt to the increase in pressure. Specific active remodeling cells and chemicals are also carried in the increased blood to the stressed area.

It is here that we have contradiction. For a bone or tendon to become stronger, it first goes through a weakening phase. The weakened structure must be taken down and replaced by a stronger structure. It is at the height of the taking down or removal phase (just before adequate rebuilding has occurred) that the system breaks down. This usually takes place at three weeks into the high stress period. A small incomplete break (fracture) of the bone or small tear of the tendon appears. See figure 12-1. If

FIGURE 12-1. *Bone scan—stress fracture*

this part is not appropriately rested, a full blown complete fracture or complete rupture of the tendon may ensue.

We must emphasize that most stress fractures and tendinitis problems are not casted. In fact, total rest only delays the rebuilding process. When you resume activity, pain recurs.

"Relative rest" best describes the sensible treatment for stress reactions, stress fractures, and tendinitis. A patient should be allowed to continue stressing the injured extremity at a painless level with specific prescribed exercises. Walking, biking, swimming, or light leg weight exercises may be substitutes for running. This approach allows the remodeling process to catch up and the tissue to become strong. Gradual resumption of full activity is allowed usually over a six to eight week

Tina, a sixteen-year-old star varsity cross country runner, came to my clinic with complaints of significant pain on the inside of both legs. The right hurt worse than the left. She had experienced aches and pains every track season in her knees, Achilles tendons, and arches of her feet.

My examination showed an area of pain and tenderness about three inches long on the inside of the lower part of her legs. She limped on the right leg. There was little swelling and no unusual warmth in the area. Her x-rays were normal. Because of her intense desire to return to her training, I ordered a bone scan to confirm a diagnosis of stress fracture versus shin splints. The bone scan showed increased blood flow to the painful area and was a stress fracture. She also had bilateral pronated feet.

Her treatment included short-term crutch use until the pain subsided. Then she started a low impact aerobic program (biking, swimming, and light weights workout) for the next three weeks. As her symptoms improved, she resumed a gradual running program on a cushioned track. She was also given a prescription for custom orthotics because of her history of stress reactions and pronated feet. She has recovered completely and is now a competitive runner in college.

period. Remember that tendons remodel just like bone and most inflamed tendons are also overstress injuries. Tendinitis also occurs more commonly in tight-muscled patients or is secondary to imbalances between muscle groups.

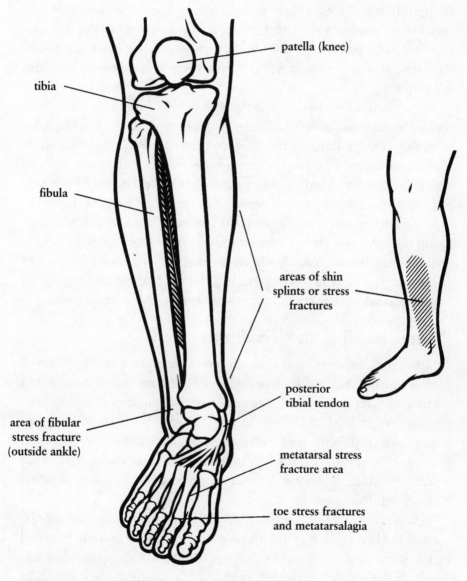

FIGURE 12-2. *Areas of stress*

ACHILLES TENDINITIS OR RUPTURE

Just in case you don't know the story behind Achilles heel, Greek mythology talks about a Greek by the name of Achilles who was a great leader and warrior. When he was a child, his mother took him by one heel and dropped him in the river Styx to make him physically invulnerable. But much to the mother's surprise, the heel held in her hand stayed dry and, therefore, was vulnerable. During the battle for Troy, he was slain by Paris who shot an arrow in Achilles' only vulnerable spot—his heel, and killed him.

In the medical profession, the Achilles tendon is the continuation of the calf muscle, and inflammation of the tendon is referred to as Achilles tendinitis. This problem is the most common tendon inflammation or injury, although any tendon (including back muscles and tendons) can be affected. Your heel cord (Achilles tendon) is the extension of the two large calf muscles—the gastrocnemius and the soleus muscles. It attaches to the back of the heel (calcaneous). The main function of this muscle group is to give you push off power (rising onto tiptoes) during walking or jumping activities. You should realize that running itself is a series of small jumps. Since the forces generated during running or jumping far exceed normal activity stress, micro-tears in this tendon are common.

Plantar Fasciitis and Tendinitis

Athletes, runners, and others active in sports are aware of the problem of plantar fasciitis (inflammation of the plantar fasciae). As we discussed in detail in chapter 8, the fascia has two important functions: to help support the longitudinal arch of the foot and provide push off power when beginning to rise on the toes. Extra stress on the fascia due to abnormal pronation eventually causes inflammation and tear away from their attachment at the heel bone. It is analogous to someone trying to pull a hunk of hair from your head.

Since there is a close functional relationship between the plantar fascia and the heel cord, it is not uncommon for both to become inflamed at the same time, resulting in Achilles tendinitis and plantar fasciitis. These are the primary instigators of rear foot pain. As discussed in chapter 8, plantar ligament strain and pain is common in the athletic population. It may stem from one severe injury or repetitive overstress injuries. The arch ligament (plantar fascia) which extends from the heel to the toe is stretched and tightened when you roll over the foot during walking or running. You can feel the ligament tighten by pulling up on your toes. It is described as a "windlass" mechanism. When stress exceeds strength, failure and symptoms occur.

For plantar fasciitis sufferers, getting up in the morning is often a chore. The classic characteristic is pain in the inflamed area when you first put pressure on the foot in the morning. After walking for several minutes, the pain goes away and normal walking with minimal discomfort resumes. Any lengthy sitting or lying idle during the day often brings back the pain once weight is again put on the foot. The culprit is plantar fascia.

Plantar fascia can torment its sufferers for years. The treatment is the same as that of acute ligament injuries. Unfortunately, the healing period may be prolonged. Surgery to release the ligament is occasionally necessary but rarely before nine to twelve months.

Symptoms of Tendinitis

Your symptoms may develop gradually or appear suddenly. If a complete rupture (total disruption) of the tendon occurs, you will experience severe pain—as if someone has hit the back of your ankle or calf with a sledgehammer. You may even look around for your attacker. Frequently, you can feel a tearing sensation and you will hardly be able to walk. You will also feel immediate weakness in the leg.

When you have tendinitis, the onset of symptoms is less abrupt and less disabling at first, but progresses if activity is continued. You may first notice a mild ache in the injured area after the activity. Most people attribute these symptoms to the "normal aches and pains of life." You may continue to overstress the injured area which will begin hurting during the activity. Some people continue their workout and try to work through the discomfort. But with continued overstress, the symptoms eventually become severe and disabling and can even lead to complete tendon rupture. This sequence of symptoms may creep over a period of weeks or even months. The "no pain, no gain" attitude to recover from injury is inappropriate.

As a general rule, the longer the symptoms have been present before treatment, the longer the recovery time. Swelling and warmth from inflammation are often present—either localized to the injured area or spread over a larger part of the limb. See figure 12-3.

Self-Help Treatment

PREVENTION is the key to self-help for shin splints and tendinitis. A proper and gradual conditioning program is highly recommended. For the novice runner, various approaches have been recommended. Proper warm-up is essential before participating in any sports activity. At rest, cold muscles are inflexible and at a higher risk of injury. Increasing the blood flow to the muscle during the initial warm-up makes it more adaptable. Moist heat application or doing some gentle jumping jacks, light jogging, or massage should take care of the warm-up phase.

The next step should be appropriate muscle tendon stretches. You should conclude the run or other sports activity with repeat stretching. It is a very important step to remember. If a mild ache occurs, the injured part should be iced down after the activity to help alleviate inflammation.

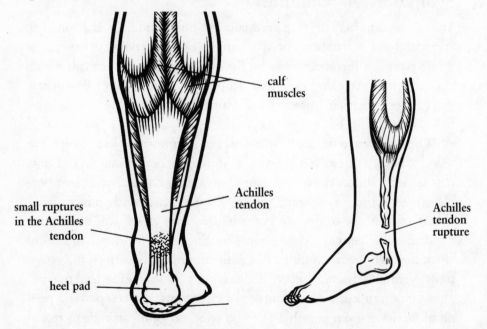

FIGURE 12-3. *Achilles tendinitis and rupture*

Important tips

The MOST important self-help advice YOU get is to recognize a developing pain and evaluate it accordingly. Some of the honest questions you should ask yourself are:

- Did I overdo it? Was it from a too rapid conditioning program, running too many miles, climbing too many hills, or exercising too many consecutive days?

- What specific motion causes my pain? Is it from jumping, landing, twisting, or from the shock of my leg hitting the ground?

- Does my technique need evaluation or coaching? Who should I see? How soon?

- Is my sports equipment faulty or worn? Are my shoes worn or do they fit poorly? Is my equipment the proper weight, length, and so on?

- Was there an environmental effect? Was the surface too hard, artificial turf, bad weather? What alternatives do I have? What could happen if I don't heed the warning signals?

A mild anti-inflammatory medicine may be used before or after the activity, but you should first diagnose your symptoms and their cause. Masking the symptoms is only prolonging and/or potentially creating a more serious problem.

"When should I see a doctor?" is a common question that is somewhat difficult to answer. No one knows your body as well as you do. As you become more mature (agewise), you can recognize and expect and even accept certain aches and pains. But any traumatic injury to joints (including sprained ankles) should be medically evaluated. Severe pain raises red flag warnings—see your doctor! Persisting bone or joint pain over two or three weeks requires further evaluation and treatment. Infections in the foot, including ingrown toe nails, should be promptly treated. In any event, if you are worried about how you feel, you should see your doctor. Remember the five harmful words in medicine—"Maybe it will go away!" Remember also RICE—Rest, Ice, Compression, and Elevation. This is good advice for any acute injury or swelling. Ice is frequently used for several weeks (post-injury) to combat swelling and inflammation. Using heat actually causes more swelling. It should not be used during the early healing phase—often not for two to three weeks. More on RICE is covered later in this chapter and in chapter 16.

I cannot overemphasize the importance of correct diagnosis. It is true that stress fractures can occur anywhere, but the most severe repercussions show up in the back (**spondylosis**) or hip (groin or thigh pain). The most common leg stress fractures are in the metatarsal bones of the forefoot and occasionally in the heel. Leg stress fractures of the tibia or fibula can occur anywhere on the bone.

Characteristically, the pain and mild swelling are on the inside of the leg bone. It is the area where "shin splints" also occur. Shin splints are a problem of overuse of the adjacent soft tissue, primarily the post-tibial tendon and adjacent bone covering (periosteum). Both shin splints and leg stress fractures are commonly associated with hyperpronation stresses. People with this problem often have inturned knee caps (femoral torsion) or flat feet which anatomically can lead to this overstress condition.

Medical Treatment

If you have a stress fracture, "relative" rest and nonpainful exercise is the best prescription. You need a physical therapist or a trainer to evaluate proper stretching and training techniques for your condition. Once you begin to walk and carry out everyday activities with no pain (no limp, and so on), then you can gradually resume running and other sports. However, resume these activities gradually and painlessly.

To differentiate a stress fracture from a shin splint or tendinitis, a bone scan may be needed. This special x-ray highlights the injured area when regular x-rays appear normal. But since shin splints and stress fractures are treated essentially the same way, the bone scan is not necessary in most cases.

A frequently prescribed medicine is NSAIDs which help combat inflammation and swelling. Although they also help relieve pain, the goal is inflammation relief so that a graduated exercise program can be resumed. Crutches are prescribed, especially in the case of a significant limp. Crutches allow proper rest of the injured part. They also protect the other joints or body parts from strain due to the stresses caused by the limp. For the acute phase, RICE is prescribed. Casts are rarely used, although sometimes for function at work, and elsewhere, a short leg cast may be needed for a brief period of time.

Treating a foot stress fracture with a stiff sole shoe or cast shoe can be very helpful. Molded cushion or semirigid orthotics are prescribed to give the sufferer better shock absorption or motion control. These devices reduce the amount of pronation or supination.

A ³/₈-inch heel lift or a higher heel shoe may be prescribed for Achilles tendinitis to help relieve stress of the tendon during normal activity.

Physical therapy should be prescribed early in the treatment of tendinitis. It generally includes the use of modalities such as electrical stimulation and a cryopump to control swelling. It is combined with progressive stretching and strengthening of the affected tendon and muscles. It is frequently extended to a home program which should be continued. See chapter 16.

Orthotics to control abnormal motions are occasionally prescribed if a shin splint or chronic tendinitis problem exists.

Surgical Treatment

Surgery is rarely necessary for tendinitis or stress fracture problems. The exception is a stress fracture to the small toe metatarsal. This bone injury is a problem because the small toe has less blood supply, heals slowly (or not at all), and may require internal fixation with a screw and/or bone graft to assist healing. Sometimes, other bones in the foot will fail to heal and require surgery. With any of these problems, you should look for underlying causes such as adjacent joint problems, misaligned bones, or weak muscles.

A tendinitis problem usually heals with appropriate medical treatment. Occasionally, the damage may be significant enough or the inflammation serious enough to make it unresponsive. Medical treatment should first be tried. Several methods of treatment may be needed to get the desired result. Surgery should be considered only after these treatments have failed. Surgery involves removing the inflamed covering over the tendon (tenosynovectomy) and then repairing the tendon. It is rarely considered before several months of conservative therapy is tried.

In cases of acute Achilles tendon rupture, there are two accepted treatments. One is casting with the foot pointed down for approximately eight weeks, followed by a course of physical therapy. The other is surgical repair used when the patient is medically healthy and is an active person. Casting or splinting is still required after surgery for approximately eight weeks. Research studies have shown that healing is slightly better with surgical repair and the chance of rerupture is less likely. See chapter 9 on flat feet for a discussion of post-tibial tendinitis.

ACUTE INJURIES

Ankle sprains and fractures are the most common injuries treated in an orthopedic clinic. Ankle sprains occur in all walks of life with all degrees of severity in an estimated two million people a year. If you have sustained an ankle injury that has pain and/or swelling, you should have medical treatment and foot/ankle x-rays should be taken. An ankle fracture must be distinguished from a sprain or ligament tear. Sometimes, a small piece of bone may be pulled off by the ligament attached to this area. Even though it is literally a fracture, it is considered a sprain with an associated avulsion injury (small piece of bone pulled off with the ligament).

Fractures

A fracture is a broken or cracked bone. It may be displaced (out of position, malangulated) or non-displaced (minimal or no angulation including stress fractures). It may be an open fracture (protruding through the skin) or a closed fracture (no skin breakage). It may also be a comminuted fracture (broken in several pieces) or a simple fracture (two fracture pieces). See figure 12-4.

When any joint is fractured, the goal is to return that joint to as nearly a normal an anatomy as possible. Even a small displacement of a joint injury will lead to future symptomatic traumatic arthritis. As a result, most ankle fractures require surgery and fixation with screws, plates, pins, or staples to try to restore normal joint anatomy. Unfortunately, even restoring this anatomy does not always prevent future arthritis. Fractures sometimes take a long time to heal (delayed healing), and

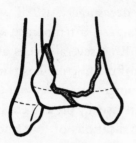

A. simple fracture (ankle)

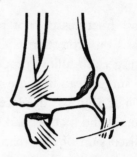

B. displaced fracture (ankle)

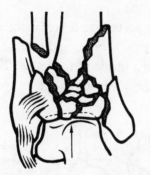

C. comminuted fracture (ankle)

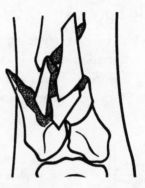

D. open fracture (broken through the skin)

FIGURE 12-4. *Types of fractures*

more rarely, they do not heal (non-union). This problem can occur with or without surgery and requires further treatment. Infection or skin healing problems are always a potential problem. The risk of infection is greater with more severe trauma, if surgery is performed, or if it is an open fracture. See chapter 11 for more details.

Heel (calcaneous) fractures often occur after you fall from a height and land on your heel. This is frequently a comminuted fracture. It is a fairly common injury and is treated in a variety of ways including bandages and crutches, casting, or surgery. In the past, attempting to fix this heel fracture was described as trying to put Humpty Dumpty back together. But with significantly improved surgical techniques and better diagnostic tools like the CAT scan and MRI, surgery of the heel has become much more successful than before and, in most cases, is the treatment of choice.

Most fractures do not require emergency surgery. RICE, with an emphasis on protection (splinting or casting), is a temporary solution with surgery to follow proper evaluation. Even several weeks after the injury, surgery can be quite successful. But if the fracture has punctured the skin or is grossly displaced, emergency surgery is carried out to clean the wound and fix the break. Antibiotics are usually prescribed. For further discussion of the treatment and complications of foot and ankle fractures, refer to chapter 14.

Ankle Sprains

When you have an ankle injury, it is important to describe the way the injury occurred. Most ankle injuries happen by twisting the ankle inward, causing a tearing of the ligaments on the outside of the ankle. This happens in 90 percent of ankle sprains. These are called inversion sprains.

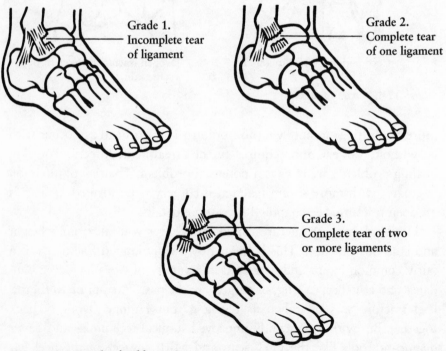

Grade 1.
Incomplete tear
of ligament

Grade 2.
Complete tear
of one ligament

Grade 3.
Complete tear of two
or more ligaments

FIGURE 12-5. *Levels of ankle sprains*

Less frequently, a pronation stress may be the cause of the ankle sprain. In such a case, the ligaments on the inside and middle of the ankle feel very tender or painful. It is important to accurately differentiate these mechanisms, because the inside ankle sprain takes much longer to heal than the more common inversion sprain.

Ankle sprains are graded as mild (1), moderate (2), or severe (3). In each grade, there is tearing of the ligament—the difference being the severity of the tear. We often see an athlete who "sprains his/her ankle" and, after treatment, returns to play in the same game. Even in a mild sprain, returning to the sport immediately carries some risk of further injury. The "risk versus gain" issue should be considered before continuing a high risk activity.

Although most ankle sprains heal with appropriate protection and treatment (on the average between two and six weeks after injury), about one-third of patients will have prolonged swelling and discomfort. This is usually secondary to developing excess scar tissue, a small, loose fragment not initially seen on x-rays, or by subtle injury to adjoining joints that was not previously detected.

Key Conditions

There are several conditions that cause prolonged ankle pain or disability:

- Additional injury—Achilles tendon rupture, fifth metatarsal (Jones) fracture, or other foot fractures.

- Scar tissue in the ankle (Wolin's sign).

- Failure of scar tissue to heal properly leading to recurrent ankle sprains.

- Tendons/muscles which are too tight and lead to repetitive ankle stress.

Medical Treatment

If you have a joint injury and swelling, you should see your doctor. x-rays are necessary to rule out fractures or dislocations and to evaluate the amount of instability.

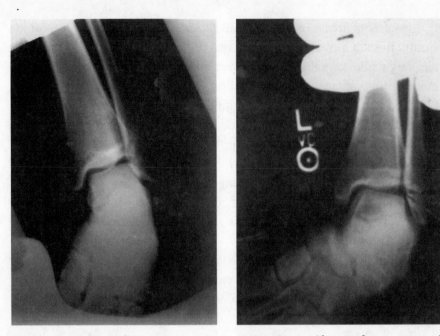

FIGURE 12-6A. *Normal stress x-ray*

FIGURE 12-6B. *Abnormal stress x-ray of left ankle. Arrow points to abnormal tilt of talus.*

RICE Treatment

Let's talk a little more about this important treatment by explaining the letters and what they mean:

R is *rest* which means crutches with limited weightbearing. It also includes protective supports like air casts, get casts, and so on, which allow a gentle up and down motion of the foot and ankle but limit twisting. Occasionally, a cast or splint is used to immediately rest the injury.

I for *ice* (NOT heat) is used for acute injury. It should be used as long as swelling persists, which may be several weeks. Ice is applied for fifteen to twenty minutes every hour for the first six to twelve hours after the injury. After that, it should be used at least several times a day. You should have a towel or other device between the ice and your skin for protection.

Another treatment for swelling control is a *cryopump*. This device is a cuff that applies cold and intermittent pressure during the acute phase of the injury. Many physical therapy departments have this device. It may be rented for home use by a simple prescription.

C stands for *compression*. Compression may be an Ace bandage, compression stockings, pump, or gel wrap. If the compression device becomes tight from swelling, it MUST be released or loosened.

E represents *elevation*, which is a critical step. The foot should be raised above the heart for the first forty-eight hours after the injury. It is very important to elevate the injured limb as much as possible until swelling is gone.

Remember that any foot or ankle that has been injured or has had surgery tends to swell inordinately because of its distance from the heart. The tendency is for blood to pool in the foot or ankle. Prolonged morbidity or disability may be avoided if swelling is controlled. It is the *most important factor* in returning the athlete to early competition.

What about physical therapy? For more severe sprains, physical therapy is usually prescribed. The therapy generally includes:

- Swelling control
- Proper muscle strengthening
- Early motion to pump fluid from the injury site
- Electrical stimulation to control swelling

Heel cord stretching is especially important. Physical therapy strengthening exercises help eliminate muscle imbalances that contribute to ankle

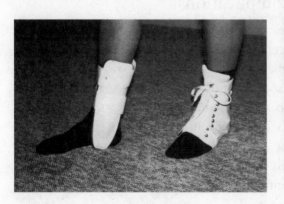

FIGURE 12-7A. *Air cast and lace-up ankle support*

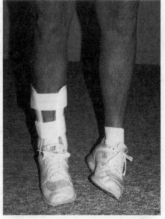

FIGURE 12-7B. *Air cast demonstrates how ankle inversion is prevented.*

sprains. As the ankle heals, coordination and speed exercises are started to include hopping on one leg, roller board balance, and response time drills. When painless full motion and ankle strength have been restored, the athlete can return to full activity. This should be carefully monitored, though, and the athlete should not start up again at "full speed" without consulting his or her doctor. Taping, a lace-up ankle support, or an elastic support is often prescribed. See chapter 16.

Surgical Treatment

Surgery is rarely indicated for an acute ankle sprain. It is performed in less than five percent of cases. But if there are recurrent ankle sprains or a sprain that does not respond to other treatment, surgery is sometimes a choice. Ankle *arthroscopy* may be recommended if the primary symptom is a painful ankle. Through small incisions, the ankle joint and surrounding soft tissue can be examined and scar tissue or small chip fractures can be removed. This procedure is performed by an orthopedic surgeon.

If the problem is recurrent ankle sprains, repair of the ankle ligaments is done (Brostrom procedure). If the ankle is highly unstable, a tendon from the outside of the ankle may be used for further support. After this procedure, casting is usually required for four to eight weeks. There is a seventy-five to eighty percent chance the patient will successfully return to previous activity levels.

Expectations and Complications

Recurrent ankle sprains mean arthritis developing in different degrees of severity. It is treated like other arthritis problems and the prognosis (long-term prediction) varies. Sometimes, after ligament repair, the ankle/hindfoot (subtalar) joints lose some motion and flexibility. You might find uneven surface walking especially troublesome. In 10 to 15 percent of cases, the ligament repair will stretch out or be only partially successful. Numbness to the top or lateral (outside) of the foot may occur after ankle surgeries. This usually does not affect the muscles or ankle function. However, it can be annoying. On rare occasions, a symptomatic neurom may occur. See chapter 7.

George, a twenty-eight-year-old avid basketball player, was referred from the emergency room with a badly swollen ankle. He was an excellent player and had played basketball for his university. He made a quick cut (turn) to the left and his right ankle twisted under him. He felt a tearing sensation and the ankle swelled quickly. Within an hour, his ankle was severely swollen and he went to the emergency room. He had a history of recurrent ankle sprains and usually wore a protective ankle brace.

Examination showed tight heel cords, a high arch, and an inverted heel. He had a common inversion injury to his ankle with a tearing of the outside ankle ligaments. Both of his ankles were unstable from previous injuries. The x-rays showed no fractures, but a gentle stress x-ray showed an unstable ankle joint.

George was treated with crutches, an air cast, NSAIDs, and told to use ice at least three times a day. He was instructed to elevate his leg as much as possible. He was sent to physical therapy for modalities to include electrical stimulation and a cryopump for swelling control and a gentle up and down range of motion exercises. He then progressed to ankle strengthening and stretching exercises. (See chapter 17 on rehabilitation.)

George recovered from his acute injury but continued to feel weakness in his ankle when he was active, despite taping and an ankle brace. The angle of his heel and his ligament injuries made him a candidate for more ankle sprains. He felt his quality of life was compromised and elected to have surgery to correct the problem. I cut and realigned his heel bone to a more stable position (osteotomy) and surgically tightened his ankle ligaments. George recovered quickly and eventually resumed playing sports. He has some mild stiffness in his ankle, but is not limited by it.

IN A NUTSHELL

Gradual and proper conditioning programs will be a real plus for your health. However, many sports injuries are the result of over-stress and overuse. Pay attention to pain, swelling, and other symptoms and see your doctor if they persist. Make sure that the sports equipment you use, including your shoes, is not worn out.

RICE is good advice for any acute injury. Controlling swelling is a sure way to return to your sport quickly

DOCTOR'S CORNER: QUESTIONS AND ANSWERS

My doctor prescribed custom orthotics for my ankle and shin splints problem. They are so expensive and my insurance won't pay for them. Are they worth it?

Custom orthotics are usually prescribed after simple over-the-counter shoe inserts and shoe modifications have been tried and failed. Custom orthotics control abnormal motions like overpronation and oversupination, and provide shock absorption or a combination of these. They are made of a variety of materials. A specialist is needed to determine the correct type for you.

Custom orthotics have been very beneficial in helping shin splints and other problems. It is important to avoid the common error of not evaluating shoes to fit these orthotics so that they can do their job.

I sprained my ankle three months ago, but it is still swollen. What should I do about it?

Thirty to forty percent of ankle sprains have some persistent swelling or other problems many months after the injury. You need to continue the ankle exercises and stretching that you learned in physical therapy and should wear your ankle support while you are active. You also need to wear proper shoes for support. Most ankle problems will resolve with time, patience, and common sense. Only rarely will scar tissue or ankle instability require surgical correction.

My son's foot was stepped on in a football game by a 250-pound lineman and it is very swollen. What should I do for him?

Acute swelling of the foot is a potential medical emergency. As the swelling gets worse, it cuts off circulation to the small muscles of the foot and, within a few hours, they can die. Get medical help right away. Even if no fracture is present, the patient needs medical help when there is progressive pain and swelling. Don't wait until the next morning, because this may be a case of muscle compartment syndrome which needs treatment.

TERMS TO REMEMBER

Achilles tendinitis: Inflammation or microscopic tears of the calf tendon.

Ankle arthroscopy: A surgical procedure, where scar tissue or small chip is removed from the ankle by an arthroscope through small incisions.

Arthroscopy: Small incision surgery using a small tube lens system that is inserted to allow visualization of the entire joint with a small camera. Small surgical instruments inserted into tiny incisions are used to perform the surgery.

Calcaneous fracture: Heel fracture.

Closed fracture: A break with no skin breakage.

Comminuted fracture: A bone broken in several places.

Displaced fracture: A fracture that is out of position.

Fracture: A small, incomplete break; a broken or cracked bone.

Inversion sprain: Twisting the ankle inward causing a tear of the ligaments on the outside of the ankle.

Open fracture: A break protruding through the skin.

Plantar fasciitis: Inflammation of the arch ligament or the plantar fascia.

Relative rest: Continuing to stress the injured extremity at a painless level.

RICE: Rest, ice, compression, and elevation; a procedure to combat swelling and inflammation.

Rupture: Complete tearing of the tendon or a ligament.

Simple fracture: A break with two fracture pieces.

Spondylosis: Stress fracture in the back of the patient.

Stress fracture: A painful reaction of bone that occurs when the stress applied to it has exceeded the bone's ability to withstand or remodel to that stress.

Tendinitis: Inflammation and/or micro-tears of a tendon or surrounding tendon sheath.

Wolin's sign: Scar tissue in the ankle after ankle sprain.

CHAPTER 13

I've Had Nail and Skin Problems on My Feet. Help!

INTRODUCTION

Infection is a constant threat to the human body. For some, infection occurs more often and lasts longer, depending on the individual's immune system, state of health, and the general environment. When it comes to foot infection, you can experience an infection anywhere on the foot, especially in areas where there is excessive moisture. This especially means the areas between your toes where moisture predominates due to sweating or lack of ventilation.

For many people, nail and skin problems are a never-ending hassle. With the threat of infection and its accompanying problems, prevention is your first line of defense. Taking proper precautions can pay dividends in the long run.

Athlete's foot is a common problem among runners, other athlete's, and people who walk a lot or stand on their feet all day. Shoes or socks made from nonbreathing material DON'T contribute to healthy, dry feet. Non-shoe wearing people have a low incidence of athlete's foot, but they are more vulnerable to secondary infection from foot lacerations (cuts) or injuries.

Athlete's foot can easily be mistaken for contact dermatitis, an allergic reaction to shoe components or other materials. A "sweaty or smelly foot" problem may also be related to foot infection, or it may be caused by an inherent tendency to perspire excessively. Whatever the cause, regular inspection of the feet and good hygiene can save you a lot of discomfort and help your feet look and stay healthy, regardless of age or occupation.

NATURAL HISTORY OF ATHLETE'S FOOT (TINEA PEDIS)

Athlete's foot is the most common fungus infection afflicting our population. In fact, ninety percent of adults have fungal involvement of their toe web spaces and ninety-five percent of these cases are asymptomatic. This problem occurs in all ages and both sexes, although it is more common in men than women. Hot humid climates, participating in athletics at all levels, use of public showers or pools, and foot trauma increase the chance of getting athlete's foot. The time elapsed from exposure to the fungus to the appearance of symptoms is anywhere from two to thirty-eight weeks. A sweaty and warm foot environment is a breeding ground for both fungus and bacteria. See figure 13-1.

If you have the milder, less draining form of infection, it is primarily a fungus. But the acute and more symptomatic infection is more likely bacterial or a combination of bacteria and fungus. With treatment, most infections clear in two to four weeks; others can take three to four months.

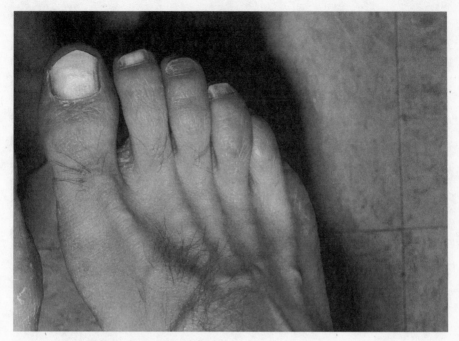

FIGURE 13-1. *Athlete's foot and nail fungus*

Symptoms: Infections

As we mentioned earlier, the most common fungus infection is found between your toes and often leads to fissure formation (skin cracking). The infected area looks scaly and whitish with no associated pain, itch, or odor. Other infections show cracking or ulcerations of the skin, itching, and odor. Redness, swelling, and pain come with severe infections. The more deep-seated skin infections have symptoms of persistent itching (pruritic).

A third variety of fungus infection appears as patchy, thickened, dry, scaly, noninflamed areas on the sole or heel of the foot. Both feet (sometimes the palm of your hand) may be afflicted. Occasionally, you may have a fungal skin infection that also involves your toenails. In particular, this infection of the sole and/or the coexistence of a fungal nail infection is quite resistant to treatment and medical evaluation, and treatment should be sought early. See figure 13-2.

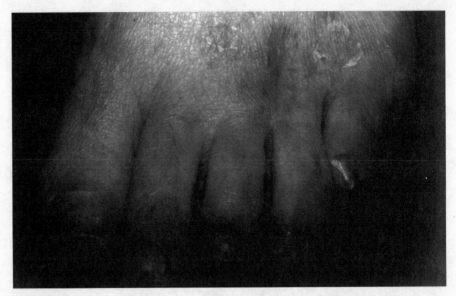

FIGURE 13-2. *Fungus of skin (tinea pedis) and nail infection (onchymyosis)*

Self-Help Treatment: Infections

What can you do about this type of uninvited "nuisance"? *Prevention* is the key word to remember. Here are some things you can do to prevent or treat fungus infections:

1. Keep your feet as dry as possible, especially after showers.

2. Wear absorbent cotton socks which are better than wool or synthetic (nylon) materials.

3. Wear nonocclusive shoes (leather) or sandals. They make it easier for your feet to breathe.

4. Do not use talc powder on your toes because it acts as an irritant and combines with moisture to promote fungal growth. Talc was recommended in the past, but no longer.

5. Use shower clogs and avoid walking or standing barefoot on public floors to avoid contamination or secondary infection.

6. If you have itching or cracking between your toes, you should apply antifungal cream twice a day. Halog, Micatin, or Desenex cream

applied to the infected area is quite effective. There are a number of other over-the-counter antifungal medicines available.

Many people make the mistake of not applying the cream long enough. When the infection clears up (or looks better) after one or two weeks, the cream is discontinued when it should be used for at least thirty days. If the infection is still present or is not responding after seven to ten days of treatment, you should see your family doctor or a dermatologist. Use the cream (not the powder) form of the medicine, if possible.

7. If you have a scaling, blistering, or macerating (seeping, ulcerating) infection on the bottom of your foot, topical creams are not effective, since they do not penetrate the skin. Stronger prescription medicine is required.

8. If you have associated toenail and foot infection, then you should see your doctor. Your nail infection won't respond to local prescriptions, because it requires stronger medicine. The infected nail is also a persistent source of infection for your skin.

9. Any redness, crusting, associated swelling, oozing, or pustules suggests that you may have a more serious infection. In this case, you should promptly see your doctor.

10. If you are a diabetic, any infection should be seen by your doctor on an emergency basis. You need appropriate medical treatment and close monitoring.

Medical Treatment

The first step in medical (versus self help) treatment is *correct diagnosis* of the infection. To identify a fungus or a bacterial infection, your doctor may take scrapings of the infected area, place them in a potassium hydroxide solution, and examine them under a microscope. He or she will also take special cultures for further study. Contact dermatitis, psoriasis, eczema, and blisters are skin afflictions that can masquerade as a fungus infection. That is the main reason for careful tests. If the first scrapings and culture studies are negative and infection is still suspected, the test should be repeated. First studies can miss the infection!

OTHER DIAGNOSES TO CONSIDER

Warts

Warts are actually a skin infection caused by a virus. Calluses, corns, and warts are commonly confused. The differences and treatments are discussed in chapter 6.

Contact Dermatitis

Contact dermatitis may be an allergic reaction to shoe materials or to chemical additives in the rubber used in shoe construction. It may also be an allergic reaction to anything your feet come in contact with like carpets, floor wax or polish, grass, fertilizers, and the like. It is diagnosed by its location, typicaly on top of your feet or toes. This allergic reaction generally involves the dorsal surfaces of both feet. There is usually crusting and oozing. When this happens, your doctor should perform allergic patch testing on your skin.

It is very rare to find contact dermatitis in the toe web spaces or on the bottom of the foot, although it can occur. See figure 13-3.

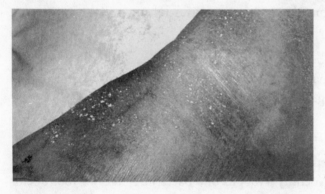

FIGURE 13-3. *Contact dermatitis*

Psoriasis

Psoriasis is a condition that shows up as a scaling eruption on several areas of the foot and other areas of the body. It is often associated with arthritis. According to one source, psoriatic arthritis develops in twenty percent of patients with psoriasis. Genetic, environmental, and infectious factors are known to trigger this condition.

Eczema

There are all kinds of foot rashes that are associated with fissuring (cracking) and maceration. Maceration is a breaking down of skin tissue that is often associated with oozing. These foot rashes are grouped into the eczema category. Dyshidrosis (a sweating abnormality), neurodermatitis with scaling or rash, as well as atopic dermatitis are examples of eczema. These conditions can be initiated by stress. These problems tend to be recurrent and/or chronic or long lasting.

Eczema is diagnosed by a process of elimination. The first step is to prepare a careful family history of the patient, perform a social and job history (stress) examination, and do appropriate testing to rule out fungus or bacterial infection or contact dermatitis. Once the correct diagnosis is determined, then the appropriate treatment follows.

Treatment

For fungus skin infection (**tinea pedis**), see self help if your condition is scaly or mildly macerating and located between the toes.

You can try multiple topical medications, but use the cream form, not aerosol sprays or powders. Any of the following prescription medications may be effective:

- Naftifine HCL (more recently introduced)
- Ciclopriox (also effective against some bacteria)
- Econazole
- Oxiconazole
- Ketoconazole
- Sulconazole
- Lotrimin and Micatin sold over the counter may also help.

It is important to massage the medication into the affected area and a few inches around it twice a day. Continue the treatment for at least thirty days. A scaly rash on the bottom of your foot does not respond to this type of treatment and will require oral medications. If topical treatment fails, an oral medicine will be prescribed.

Griseofulvin Ultramicrosize (250 to 500 milligrams taken twice a day) is prescribed for most fungus infections, with the exception of candida infection. Ketoconazole (200 milligrams daily) is used for this fungus, but is associated with more side effects. See toenail infection.

Bacterial infections are treated with antibiotics based on the culture results. Keflex or Dicloxicillin are used initially to treat the most common staphylococcus (staph) or streptococcus (strep) bacterial infections until the culture results are available in usually twenty-four hours.

Contact dermatitis and eczema should be treated by first finding out the cause of the allergy or identifying the precipitating cause. You should first treat an oozing or crusty dermatitis with warm soaks twice a day; then carefully dry the area. If itching or burning symptoms are significant, cold compresses, calamine lotion, or topical benadryl may be tried. Burows solution (or twenty-nine percent acetic acid solution) applied for twenty minutes two to four times a day may also be used. This may not be any more effective than plain warm soaks to dry up the affected area.

Once the oozing has stopped, you can massage one percent hydrocortisone cream into the area twice a day. If your symptoms are severe, your doctor may prescribe a short course of prednisone (cortisone) taken orally.

Warts (virus infection) and calluses specifically discussed in chapter 6 should not be mistaken for other common skin problems.

Less Common Skin Problems

There are less common skin problems like viruses (herpes), mycobacterium (an atypical T.B.-like bacteria found in brackish and contaminated water), or folliculitis (small pustules) occurring in infected hair follicles. Treatment of these conditions is effective, but your doctor must first make the correct diagnosis before taking appropriate measures.

Smelly feet (**bromhidrosis**) is a symptom (not a diagnosis of a problem) you may have. It is a major complaint with some patients. Excess sweating may be genetic, the result of low grade infection, stress related, or simply caused by occlusive footwear that does not allow proper foot breathing. Trying to find the cause is important, as your sweaty feet can be treated.

A medicated foot powder may be applied daily or Drysol (25 percent aluminum chloride in anhydrous ethyl chloride), which requires a prescription, should be applied at night. This can be followed by covering the foot with a plastic occlusive wrap which is washed off in the morning. DO NOT apply Drysol to cracked or crusty areas of the foot. After the condition has cleared, the medication and treatment should be used only as needed. A dermatologist may be required if your sweaty feet become a chronic and significant problem.

Blisters

Blisters are fluid-filled sacs that result from friction between the skin and another surface, such as the shoe. It is the body's initial response to friction and pressure. If left untreated, they can swell and become infected, causing severe pain with every step.

Although many people consider blisters a "minor" discomfort, others, like professional dancers or athletes, view them as catastrophic. They can be quite disabling, making walking a painful chore. Regardless of the shoes you wear or posture of your foot, it is difficult to protect your feet entirely from blisters.

Self-Care

Prevention is your first line of defense. Here are some general precautions you can take to prevent blisters or stop them from progressing:

- Wear properly fitting shoes. Abnormal shoe play (too much foot movement in the shoe) or constricting shoes are the prime causes of blisters.

- Make sure your socks fit. Socks that are too small or too large can be a problem. In some respects, a very thin sock or no sock at all in a running shoe actually decreases friction by allowing a better shoe fit.

- Early in the sports season, when starting a new sport or changing to a more stressful activity, wearing extra socks can give your feet greater protection. This is especially important when you have soft skin on your feet.

- To decrease friction, try rubbing Vaseline into the shoe or over your skin in areas of excess stress. This can really make a difference when there are demands on your feet.

- Once you have a blister, your first goal is to prevent further injury to the area. Try hard not to remove the skin over the blister. The right treatment is to puncture the edge of the blister with a flame-sterilized needle after cleaning the skin with alcohol. Place adhesive tape directly over the affected area to give it protection from infection. You must leave the tape on until it comes off on its own

- If the protective covering of skin over the blister is gone, you should clean the area thoroughly with peroxide or soap and water. Use Bacitracin ointment, followed by a protective dressing (doughnut pad or gauze pad). Then be careful to wear proper shoes to relieve the pressure on the area. When some of the discomfort is gone, expose the blister to the air and avoid pressure. If the blister becomes inflamed and painful, see your doctor. *Do not* risk an infection.

NAIL PROBLEMS

Toenail infections are not uncommon, regardless of age or sex. If your toe has ever been stepped on or hit by a heavy object, you know how uncomfortable that can be. First, there is pain, then a stinging sensation. Sometimes the skin under the nail becomes red or swollen, the symptom of an acute nail infection that is frequently related to an ingrown toenail. If left untreated, the nail could turn black—an ugly sight.

Trimming your toenail is a procedure you cannot afford to overlook. You should trim your nail straight across, not down into the margin which could result in a "nail spike" and likely inflammation. Clippers with straight edges are best for toenail trimming.

Unfortunately, when the edge of your nail cuts and presses into the flesh, you have an ingrown toenail. Some people are born with ingrown toenails. When outside pressure is applied by shoes or an injury, these nails become inflamed and infected. This can progress to a red streaking on the foot or leg, a forewarning of a more severe body infection.

People with mechanical abnormalities of their toes like bunions or mallet toes can expect problems. These abnormalities push one toe into adjacent toes, the floor, or shoes which can cause infection in the toenails. Cutting the toenail too short is enough to injure the underlying tissue or cause the nail growth to curve into the skin. Once this happens you can expect toenail infection. The culprit is often improper nail care. As we grow older, especially with diminishing eyesight, mobility, and coordination, proper nail care becomes difficult, if not impossible to manage.

The elderly, diabetics, and patients with vascular or kidney disease are at special risk and should seek help with nail care. For this category of people, infection is potentially disastrous and not worth the risk. If you have diabetes, psoriasis, thyroid conditions, and other metabolic problems, the risk of nail infection is also higher.

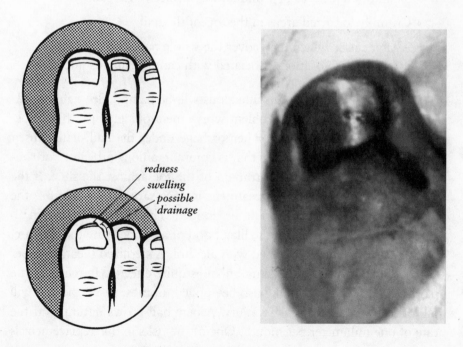

FIGURE 13-4. *Normal toenail and ingrown toenail.*

Symptoms

Improper nail care, poorly fitting shoes (narrow toe box), nail disease, or deformed toes can lead to acute or repetitive nail trauma. The tissues around the nail become red, swollen, painful, and sometimes draining. This may be a recurrent problem or only a one-time episode.

Fungus nail infection is as common as athlete's foot. It is normally unrelated to any symptoms and is more common in men than women. This type of infection often shows up in warm, moist situations such as wearing occlusive shoes, living in a humid environment, and the like. A fungus infected nail may show any of the following symptoms:

- Yellowing of the nail
- Separation of the nail plate from its bed
- Nail thickening
- Small discrete areas of white on the surface of the nail
- Crumbly localized areas in the top of the nail
- A later phase which may cover the whole nail with a yellow or greenish discoloration associated with candida fungus infection

Occasionally, these fungus infections will be painful. See figure 13-2.

There is one other nail problem worth mentioning. It is a black toenail (**subungual hematoma**) or hemorrhage under the nail plate caused by a crushing injury to the toe that is common among athletes. For runners, it is caused by repeated trauma of the toe against the shoe. If the condition is not painful, no treatment is necessary. If it is painful, the fluid under the black nail should be drained. This should be done in an emergency room because of the likelihood of an underlying toe fracture. The nail area should be cleaned with alcohol. A sterilized (heated) paper clip designed to perforate the nail plate is quite effective in relieving the pain. Sterile dressings should also be applied. In most cases, the nail will fall off a few weeks after the injury. A new nail grows naturally at the rate of one millimeter per month. One of the risks in this replacement is that the nail may grow abnormally.

Self-Help Treatment

"To treat or not to treat fungal infections?" that is the question. Your case may be isolated or involve multiple toenails. Medical treatment at best takes a long time and is expensive. Fifty percent or more of the time, it is unsuccessful. The side effects of the medicine should also be assessed. Refer to the self-help section for athlete's foot, since the same preventive measures hold true for fungus infections of the nails.

If a symptomatic or significant skin infection is also present, then a more aggressive medical treatment (with medical supervision) is required. For mild forms of fungus infection, simply scraping the nail and applying an over-the-counter topical antifungal medication may work. The treatment could take six to twelve months and still have a high failure rate. You should seek medical advice before taking such lengthy treatment.

Prevention is key to ingrown toenail problems. The course of treatment depends on the severity of the infection. If your toenail condition is mild (slight redness and no drainage), you can use moist soaks and eliminate pressure on the inflamed toe by clearing a hole in your shoe, wearing sandals, or fitting a protective toe cap. You should gently elevate and trim the nail in the affected area. If symptoms continue for more than a few days or become more severe, you should seek medical help.

For acute toe infections with significant swelling or redness and drainage, the next step is medical treatment. Remember, there is no such thing as a mild infection if you are a diabetic.

Medical Treatment

In medical treatment, the first step is proper diagnosis. A culture is taken to distinguish between bacterial infections (staph or strep) and fungus infections. The infected nail is scraped with a drop of ten to twenty percent potassium hydroxide. Then, a cover slip is gently heated and examined under a microscope to confirm the diagnosis. Prolonged treatment with oral medicines should not be started until after the diagnosis. Cultures should be obtained for both fungus and bacterial infections.

There are a number of topical antifungal medicines that can be used to prevent the fungus from spreading. They are the same medicines prescribed for tinea pedis.

For more symptomatic or significant infections, oral medicine (with or without a topical medicine) may be used. The most common medicine is Griseofulvin Ultramicrosize (250-500 milligrams) used twice a day. This treatment takes six to twelve months or longer. Candida infection does not respond to this medicine and requires Ketoconazole (200 milligrams daily) for twelve or more months.

Side Effects

There are several side effects of the following medicines that you should be aware of:

Medicine	Side effects
1. Griseofulvin	Headaches, nausea, gastrointestinal stomach upsets which may last a few days. Liver toxicity and low blood platelets are rare. Checking blood chemistries and a complete blood count every three months while on this treatment is recommended.
2. Ketoconazole	Greater incidence of kidney, liver, and blood toxicity. Nausea, vomiting, abdominal pain, itching, diarrhea, headaches, dryness, and sleepiness may occur but are less severe.

You must use oral medication until the nail shows no evidence of infection and has grown out. This takes six to twelve months. During this period and in follow up, you should apply anti-fungal medicine to the nail daily for an indefinite time to prevent recurrence.

Surgical Treatment

If medical treatments have failed or if your nail problem is acute or recurrent, the next level of treatment is nail surgery. For the acute ingrown toenail, removal of some or all of the nail and treatment with antibiotics is indicated. If the nail is deformed or there is toe deformity (like a bunion), then surgical correction of the problem should be considered.

If your nail problem is chronic, permanent removal of the nail and the nail growth cells may be necessary. This can be performed by using a chemical (phenol) which kills the growth cells, or by using surgical scraping. These procedures can be performed in the doctor's office with appropriate surgical preparation.

Occasionally, the tip of the toe and nail are surgically removed. This is rarely necessary unless other surgical treatments have failed. With any of these surgical treatments, a small portion of the nail can grow back and require another removal.

Nail surgery is performed by numbing the toe locally; there is minimal surgical risk. If the nail is removed because of resistant fungus infection, continued use of topical antifungal medicine should be followed until the new nail has grown out. Griseofulvin is frequently prescribed, as well. Remember that there is no guarantee of success or improvement with surgery. In rare cases, the condition might be made worse.

IN A NUTSHELL

Scaling or maceration between your toes is a fungus infection until proven otherwise. Allergic foot reactions may look like fungus, but you will commonly find them on the tops of both feet (a mirror image).

Fungus can also infect your toenails. Although these nails are cosmetically unattractive, they are rarely symptomatic. Treatment is usually unnecessary and often unsuccessful. If you have any infection associated with redness, pus draining, or extreme pain, you should consider it an emergency and seek medical evaluation quickly.

Bacterial infections need to be diagnosed and treated with antibiotics.

DOCTOR'S CORNER:
QUESTIONS AND ANSWERS

I have had toenail and fingernail fungus on and off for over a year. What am I doing wrong?

Obviously, fungus prevention is too late. The main error patients make is to stop using antifungal medicine too soon. They tend to stop after seven to ten days when the symptoms improve. You should use the cream, not powder form, of antifungal medicine for thirty days. If your fungus isn't much improved, you need to see your doctor. A stronger pill form of medicine may be required.

I have had a long history of ingrown toenails on my left big toe. Can this be prevented?

Nail care is very important. Your toenails need to be cut straight across and not too short. You may need professional nail care, as infected ingrown toenails can be serious. You also need to wear shoes with a wide enough toe box to avoid putting pressure on your toes/toenails. I would suggest seeing your doctor about this problem.

TERMS TO REMEMBER

Athlete's foot: A fungal infection of the foot, usually found on the sole between the toes or the sole of the foot.

Blister: A fluid-filled sac that appears as a result of friction.

Bromhidrosis: A term meaning smelly feet.

Contact dermatitis: Allergic reaction to shoe materials or chemical additives in the rubber.

Dyshidrosis: Excessive sweating tendency.

Maceration: A breaking down of skin tissue—often associated with oozing.

Psoriasis: A condition that shows up as a scaling eruption on several areas of the foot.

Subungual hematoma: Hemorrhage under the nail plate

Tinea pedis: Fungus skin infection.

Wart: A thickened, painful area of skin often mistaken for a callus. It is caused by a virus.

CHAPTER 14

Industrial/Occupational Foot Problems

INTRODUCTION

In today's highly industrialized society, occupational foot problems and injuries are an everyday occurrence. According to recent statistics from the National Safety Council, over 100,000 cases of occupationally related foot and toe injuries occur in the United States each year. This represents approximately 4 percent of all work-related injuries at an estimated cost of $2.5 billion in medical and nonmedical expenses.

Foot and ankle injuries in the workplace can be costly to employee and employer. So, safety measures taken to alleviate such injuries are essential. Doctors and organizations are now working together to enforce safety standards and ensure an injury-free work environment.

Only 17 percent of these were direct medical costs. The rest represented lost wages and insurance/administrative costs.

According to recent data from the Occupational Injury Surveyance System used by Rush Presbyterian St. Luke's Medical Center in Chicago, 58.4 percent of foot injuries were the result of being struck by an object. The rest were slips and falls, being struck against another object, or caught in, under, and between various obstructions. These injuries were suffered by all occupational groups.

There are several high-risk situations for foot and ankle injuries:

- Jobs requiring extensive *manual material handling* or vehicular operation such as fork lift trucks, crane and machine operation, construction work, and manufacturing and metal work seem to have the most serious foot and ankle injuries.

- *Youth and inexperience* seem to favor work-related accidents. Nearly half of 990 workers reporting foot injuries were between twenty and thirty years of age.

- *Summer months* (June, July, August) represent a peak in the incidence of work-related foot and ankle injuries. In contrast, the lowest frequency was reported during winter months.

- *Men* represent eighty-three percent of all occurrences, probably because most of the injuries occur in heavy labor.

- Most injuries occur on *Mondays,* with Friday mornings being the "safest" period of the week. Most of the accidents also peak just before lunch and again late in the afternoon, probably when workers' concentration levels begin to drop.

- *Lack of instruction* in the use of safety shoes and other safety measures contributes to work injuries. For instance, one study reports seventy-one percent of those reporting foot and ankle injuries did not receive any instruction about prevention.

- *Medical conditions* have been known to increase the risk of injury, including diabetes, peripheral vascular disease, degenerative arthritis, and congenital foot problems. This is why regular checkups can contribute to a healthier and safer work environment.

SPECIFIC AREAS OF OCCUPATIONAL INJURY

Ankle

The ankle joint is the most common place in the legs to suffer industrial injuries. Simply tripping over an object, slipping on a wet or slick surface, or direct trauma are the most frequent causes. A vast majority of these injuries are ankle sprains and soft tissue injuries, with only thirteen percent related to fractures.

As we discussed in chapter 12, there are degrees of severity in this commonly injured joint. Most of the injuries are treated with a protective aircast or ankle support and aggressive rehabilitation. Crutches are used for one to two weeks to avoid limping and to keep from straining other areas of the body. With these milder sprains, most people are able to return to work within four to seven days, and no persisting disability should be anticipated. Light duty, however, is prescribed for three to six weeks.

The more severe sprains present a more significant industrial problem. Most of them are treated with a cast or protective splinting. On occasion, surgery is an option for the most severe ankle sprain. Casting is usually continued for four to six weeks. You can expect marked swelling with more severe sprains and at least a week's absence from work for RICE treatment. If the patient is able to get light duty, there should be no problem returning to the workplace.

In the event the injury is to your right driving leg and you are wearing a cast, you can anticipate difficulty getting to and from work. When the cast is removed, wearing an aircast, lace-up Swedo, or lace-up Rocket Sock support will be needed for an additional four to six weeks. Returning to any kind of heavy work does not occur much before three months, and sometimes even longer. This means a good rehabilitation program is important to expedite the return of normal ankle function and strength.

Ankle Fractures

Like all other joint fractures, ankle fractures should be reduced or put back in place as close to the normal anatomy as possible. For this reason, the majority of ankle fractures require surgery with pins, plates, or screws to fix the bones in the reduced position. Post-operatively, the patient is usually protected with casts, splints, or a brace immobilization device. This device may be taken off periodically to enable the worker to move the ankle up and down, and help stimulate better cartilage and joint healing. The usual casting period ranges between six and ten weeks, followed by limited weight bearing for an additional three to six weeks. An ankle support is usually prescribed for several months for this type of injury after the cast has been removed.

The severity of the ankle fracture indicates how successful recovery can be. If the broken bone has protruded through the skin (open fracture/dislocation), there is a 25 to 40 percent chance of infection with or without surgery. Even with normal healing, light duty can be anticipated for six to nine months. Skin healing may also be a problem.

With ankle fractures, there is a significantly increased chance of developing arthritis. If the joint were reduced satisfactorily with or without surgery, there is still a chance that arthritis will occur in 8 to 14 percent of the cases. On the other hand, if the ankle is not adequately reduced, or put back in near perfect position, the chances are 30 to 40 percent. With open fraction and dislocations, the risk is even greater.

Although ankle arthritis is not uncommon after ankle fractures, functional limitations vary a great deal. Some people do not develop symptomatic arthritis for many years. At that time, it is only gradual in onset and not very limiting. Other people develop arthritis quickly, often within a year of the injury, and then become progressively disabled. This disability may require further surgery to include arthroscopic joint cleaning or ankle fusion, and there is still a chance that arthritis will occur.

With ankle injuries, the anticipated limitations include difficulties in pushing off with the foot, squatting, climbing ladders or stairs, and twisting maneuvers or working on uneven ground.

Metatarsals and Midfoot Injuries

Trauma to the forefoot is usually caused by a direct blow or a forceful turning in of the foot. The severity again varies from minor soft tissue sprains to severe crushing injuries which are associated with massive swelling and multiple fractures.

Unfortunately, many of the "minor" sprains of the midfoot and fore-foot are not taken seriously. Pain or swelling in the midfoot area raises "red flags" and should be carefully evaluated by knowledgeable medical personnel. A dislocation or partial dislocation has often gone back in place, and the x-rays look normal even though the sprain is severe. Even without fracture, these injuries are treated with casts and crutches for at least six to eight weeks. Surgery is frequently required.

Protective shoes (rocker sole) and cushioned insoles are prescribed later in treatment. Pain frequently lasts for a long time after these injuries, and arthritis develops in thirty to sixty percent of the cases. With this Lisfranc or forefoot sprain, a prolonged recovery time of at least six months can be expected. The potential may be a permanent partial disability. Isolated fractures of the metatarsal bones can also occur, but the limitations resulting from these injuries are usually not long lasting. The bones will heal with protected casting and light duty in three to four months. Surgery may be required if the metatarsal fracture is significantly displaced and causes weight-bearing pressure or a prominence.

Crush Injuries

Extensive crush injuries often affect the forefoot and midfoot. This type of injury may or may not be associated with a fracture; yet it is one of the most disabling injuries that a worker can have. A foot struck by a heavy object or caught by a moving one can swell severely and progressively. Pain also persists in spite of adequate splinting or protection. This condition may require emergency surgery to relieve the pressure, and some permanent impairment should be anticipated. The persisting pain syndrome or reflex sympathetic dystrophy is particularly common after this kind of injury. See chapter 7 for a discussion of RSD.

Toes

Toe injuries are usually caused by heavy objects falling onto the front area of the worker's foot or shoe. This type of injury may also occur when the worker jams his/her foot into an immovable object. Fortunately, steel toe caps or shoes have reduced the incidence of toe injuries. For toe fractures, there is no specific treatment required other than a short course of buddy taping (taping one toe to the other) and early ambulation in a protective shoe. See figure 14-1. Loss of work time should only be one or two days. With adequate shoe wear, the worker should return to normal function within a week or two.

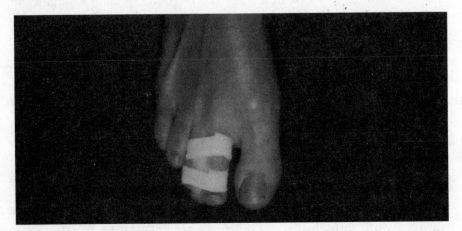

FIGURE **14-1.** *Buddy taping for toe injury*

An often underappreciated injury is a sprain or fracture of the great toe. This is commonly caused by a hyperextension or bending up of the toe toward the ankle. It results either in a small fracture or a tear of the ligament in the big toe joint. As previously discussed, the large toe is a major weight bearing area of the foot which contributes in a significant way to push off. Even though there may not be a fracture, this injury tends to remain swollen for months and long-term disability can occur. Professional football players are particularly prone to this type of injury, as artificial turf tends to bend the toe up excessively. This is a turf toe injury. Resuming play can take six to eight weeks or longer.

Heels

The heel is the first area of the leg to strike the ground while walking, running, or taking part in weight bearing activities. Trauma to the heel can be caused by chronic stress and includes injury to the heel pad, the ligament inserting into the heel, or irritation of the nerves around the heel bone. This subject is discussed in chapter 8.

B arry, a middle-age maintenance worker, was injured on the job while moving a heavy file cabinet. He was not wearing safety shoes. The cabinet crushed his left foot which began to swell alarmingly. He was sent to the emergency room where x-rays were taken. No fractures were present, but his foot continued to swell and caused him a lot of pain. The emergency room doctor admitted Barry to the hospital and called me.

I performed a needle pressure test and discovered that he had severely elevated pressures in his foot which were inhibiting circulation. Soon his foot became numb. Barry requested emergency surgery. Several incisions were made in his foot to relieve pressure. The wounds were left open for five days because of continuous swelling and then closed, requiring partial grafts.

Barry was discharged and gradually allowed to become ambulatory with the use of crutches. He did motion exercises and kept improving, although he continued to have nerve pain (numbness and burning) from the trauma injury. He has returned to light duty and is improving, though he will have a permanent disability.

Barry's company instituted a safety program and now requires the use of safe, protective shoes.

Crush injuries are serious with many potential complications. They require prompt, aggressive treatment.

Falls from some height are frequently associated with heel bone (calcaneous) fractures. These include severe injuries to the heel pad, the tendons around the bone, and the hindfoot and midfoot bones. In the past, the outlook was poor for an employee's recovery and return to work. Surgeries were unsuccessful and were compared to putting an eggshell back together. But now, with improved surgical techniques and swelling control methods, many heel fractures can be successfully corrected.

This injury can cause fractures of both heels, the back, knee, or hip. There is a related chance of fracturing one of the elbows used in trying to prevent the impact of the fall. Functional long-term limitations can be anticipated after this injury. In a recent report, however, approximately

75 percent of people with these injuries were operated on and returned satisfactorily to their work place. Special shoes and orthotic inserts are often required.

Arthritis development is not uncommon after this type of injury and often requires repeat surgery to fuse the affected joints. When limitation of the hindfoot joints occurs, walking on uneven ground, climbing, and twisting maneuvers are particularly limited. In one report, two-thirds of the patients with this injury did not reach maximum medical improvement for two to three years, while another 25 percent took up to six years.

OTHER INJURIES

Punctures

Soles

Puncture wounds from nails or other sharp objects are the most frequent causes of injuries to the sole of the foot. A tetanus injection, aggressive cleaning of the wound, and antibiotics are the normal treatment. Antibiotics are used only if the wound appears infected.

Burns

Burns occur when hot metal fragments fall inside a boot, or when molten metal is spilled into the top of a boot or around the tongue of an unprotected shoe (e.g, workers in foundries). Electrical injuries can cause severe burns to the feet. Spills of hot water or wet cement, which has high lime content, will produce serious burns. Minor superficial burns take four to six weeks to heal, while severe burns can affect all the tissues down to the bone and may even require amputation.

High pressure water injection or injection of toxic chemicals to the feet can cause special types of injuries. On the surface, they may look quite benign, but actually cause extensive soft tissue destruction and also can result in amputation. A water gun can produce a pressure of 10,000 pounds per square inch, an indication of the massive soft tissue injuries that such a device can inflict.

Reflex Sympathetic Dystrophy Syndrome (RSD)

RSD has been covered in chapter 7. This devastating problem occurs mainly after a crush injury to the ankle and foot. What really triggers it is not known, but it appears related to the autonomic or sympathetic nerve system. These nerves are put into overdrive, causing a deregulation of the blood vessels of the foot. Initially, the foot is cool and bluish in color and perspiration may be excessive. In a few weeks to a few months, the foot becomes warm, flushed, and dry. Eventually, skin becomes thin, hair gets sparse, and the foot becomes swollen and brawny.

For best results, this disease should be recognized early and treated aggressively. Pain is frequently out of proportion to the injury. The physician should be sensitive to and recognize the problem through the index of suspicion.

Treating RSD includes aggressive physical therapy. RSD blocks are performed by injecting an anesthetic into the back nerves. Disability often persists for three to six months, and even longer. The sufferer can expect long-term pain to continue.

WHY WE NEED A SYSTEM OF WORKER'S COMPENSATION?

For centuries, it has been recognized that workers need protection from unforeseen injuries on the job. Even the pirates in the early 1700s had a system of "payoff" for loss of a body part in "pieces of eight." Loss of an arm, for example, was equated to 600 pieces of eight or roughly $120,000 in 1994 U.S. dollars. In 1911, Wisconsin was the first state to enact a binding compensation law. Other states quickly followed, with benefits centering around wage loss and medical expense benefits. When these were accepted, the employee surrendered the right to sue for on-the-job injuries.

By 1949, all states had compensation systems that did not require contributions from employees. The advantage to the employee was much more prompt payment of entitlements and the elimination of so-called contributory negligence (fault of the employee). Eighty-six percent of the workforce now falls under workers compensation. The system does not include farmers, domestics, and those workers in firms of less than three employees.

Compensation Goals

There are several goals that a compensation system tries to achieve:

- Fair and prompt benefits to injured workers and their families.
- Single approach to settling personal injury suits.
- Reduce burden to other charities for caring for injured workers.
- Eliminate trials, lawyers, and witnesses.
- Safety and rehabilitation in the workplace.
- Safety and prevention through research.

These are all valuable goals, although they are difficult to administer.

Doctor's Role

Physicians are systematic in their approach to treating physical ailments. They base decisions on medical findings. In the past, medical schools and post-training programs did not emphasize how to determine disability beyond medical ailments. This evaluation incorporates not only physical ability losses, but also psychological, social, and vocational functions that are much more difficult to quantify.

The AMA Guide to the Evaluation of Permanent Impairment is the standardized reference used by physicians and evaluators to determine physical losses. It does not, however, consider other factors. The doctor is only part of a team that determines the permanent or temporary limitations of the patient based on medical evaluations. The team should be well versed in occupational and compensation laws and sensitive to the problems of injured workers.

How Can the System Be Improved?

There are several ways in which I feel the compensation system can be improved:

- *Creating doctor-worker-employee relationship.* Some organizations are creating industrial or occupational medicine clinics. Through these groups, employers are contracting to care for injured employees. This relationship allows prompt communication with the treating medical facility and direct expressions of concern about the injured worker to the physician. This way, the doctor can better understand the worker's job requirements and recommend appropriate limited duty to fit the job.

  Unfortunately, there are occasions when an employee is placed on full disability, though in fact he has many functional capabilities. In this case, there are no winners. The employer is without a worker and the employee has too much time on hand to develop fears and anxieties. As a result, the cost to the system can be excessive.

- *Using occupational medicine specialists.* This is a group of physicians especially trained to:

  - Evaluate and recognize disability.

  - Conduct independent medical evaluations to eliminate the bias of doctor-patient relationships.

  - Oversee functional capacity evaluations (evaluating specific ailments as they relate to the worker's job).

  - Oversee work hardening or conditioning programs to teach workers how to relieve pain, pace themselves, and restore self confidence.

  - To be well versed in compensation and disability laws.

  - Conduct epidemiology studies evaluating specific work environments and a relationship to disease and injury.

  - Assist in developing safety measures when, appropriate, to protect the employee.

- *Using safety engineers.* Many firms now have safety engineers to recognize unsafe practices and enforce preventive measures to minimize or eliminate injuries on the job. They also oversee safety management programs and conduct safety education programs to promote health and safety at work.

- *Establishing ergonomic centers.* This is a nationwide attempt to design desks, chairs, lighting, computer screens, and the like to human comfort and worker tolerance. These centers continue to measure the individual's functional abilities with safety and effectiveness on the job as the major goal.

- *Adding and utilizing vocational rehabilitation counselors.* These specialists are well trained in evaluating the patient's capacities. Their goal is to return the patient to full function. Their target clients are workers who have had prolonged impairments. Counselors also assist as a liaison among the employer, employee, and doctor to find the worker comparable and satisfactory employment.

- *Providing on-site rehabilitation exercise facilities.* This is a growing trend that has been adopted in a few work environments. The company sets up an appropriate exercise/rehabilitation environment at the job site with a physical therapist or personal trainer to work with the injured employee. The main advantage of this system is less time lost in secondary travel to and from rehabilitation facilities. It also keeps the worker in the workplace. The image of an "I care" atmosphere between employee and employer means better morale and loyalty to the employer, and improved alertness, endurance, and fewer injuries in the long run.

Maintaining the Work Environment

Perhaps the most effective approach to safety is a well-designed work environment. Safety equipment gives employees a sense of security on the job and a basis for regular attendance and productivity. The most crucial step in building safety into equipment is to design features that make it very difficult for the employee to be injured. For example, most modern electric grinders have guards to protect the eyes from flying metal dust or particles.

In controlling the work environment, protective gear is a must in most shops. For example, an electrician forgot one day to wear his boots. He climbed an aluminum ladder to check a loose wire on company premises. The high tension wire's powerful current jolted him off the ladder, resulting in a broken wrist and pelvis.

Recommendations

There are a number of steps that the doctor and the employer must take to ensure a safe and injury-free environment. Doctors should recognize that rarely is the worker totally disabled. Understanding the worker's job requirements in light of the existing safety equipment is also important. Therefore, when an employee has made satisfactory progress and is ready to return to work, the employer should be informed of worker readiness quickly to avoid unnecessary loss of work time.

In terms of the employer's role, several steps should be considered:

- Establish viable communication with the treating physician. This type of relationship should promote strong ties between the doctor and the organization and save lost work hours in the interim.

- Establish a fitness reward program and ensure that safety programs are instituted.

- Introduce educational courses that stress good body lifting and sitting techniques. Conducting mental stress-relieving sessions and rewarding safe practices and safety suggestions can also be helpful.

- Establish light-duty positions to allow the employee to return to work promptly and safely. Sometimes, reducing work hours is sufficient, depending on the injury.

- Offer carpools and other services that allow newly recovered workers to get to and from work on time.

- Offer courses in general safety practices at work and at home. With more work hours lost from injuries at home (lawnmower injuries, falling off ladders, and so on) than at work, such courses can pay off in the long run.

In addition to these steps, several preventive measures should be taken:

- Evaluate the surface or type of floor. Rubber matting in areas of work that require prolonged standing significantly decreases joint stress and work time lost.

- Inspect floors regularly for flaws (bumps, cracks, or uneven surfaces) to eliminate avoidable accidents or injuries.

- Check for and remove hazards such as spills, sharp objects on floors, electrical cords, wires, and the like.

- Encourage employees to participate in fitness programs and help them recognize that function (work) with protection is good for their health.

These measures make for a happier, more productive, accident-free work place.

How Important Is Safety Footwear?

The incidence of foot and ankle injuries can be significantly reduced by the universal use of "safety" shoes and implementing a safety program at work. A well-designed safety boot should prevent ankle injuries by reducing the risk of slips and falls. In order to be "slip-resistant", the soles of any safety footwear have to be soft and with a prominent tread design. Worn safety boots offer little antislip protection because of the loss of tread and the hardening of the sole material. The antislip policy can be further reinforced by the use of abrasive paints, rubber matting, or industrial carpeting. It is easy to understand that leaving high cut boots open at the top (unlaced) will not offer any protection against ankle injuries. Spilled hot water, metal, or other chemical substances also gain access to the foot and ankle more easily when the boot is not laced.

The metatarsal area (forefoot) should be protected by a metatarsal shield that must meet rigid specifications. This shield should be wide enough to protect the entire metatarsal area and overlap the toe cap of the shoe. Quick release shoes with metatarsal guards are recommended, especially for foundry workers and those in the pulp and paper industry.

Since the introduction of steel toe caps, toe injuries have fallen dramatically. The current standard requirements in the U.S. ask for an impact protection of seventy-five foot/pounds. This calculation is based on the average weight of the falling object and the height from which this object falls. To meet present industrial needs, some advocate steel toe caps that protect against an impact of 112 foot/pounds. More recently, plastic toe caps were introduced, which offer the advantage of being lighter and just as strong as the steel toe cap.

Puncture wounds to the sole can be prevented by the use of steel insoles. In fact, sole injuries have dropped dramatically since the introduction of protection against sole penetration.

Safety shoes currently come in a wide variety of sizes and styles, so there is no real reason why workers in affected industries should not wear them. Some studies report that women are less likely to wear such protective shoes because of their style, weight, or size. See figure 14-2.

Alternatively, wearing safety shoes or boots is not without problems. According to one study, ninety-one percent of the subjects wearing safety shoes reported one or more foot problems. Of those interviewed, sixty-five percent said that the shoes were excessively hot and caused fungal infection, rashes, and skin breakdowns. Under these circumstances, wearing cotton socks or stockings would certainly diminish the incidence of skin problems. The inflexible soles were the focus of complaints by fifty-two percent of those included in the study. Controlling the accelerator and brake pedals of a vehicle, climbing ladders, and crawling into confined spaces were more difficult because of inflexible shoes. Forty-seven percent of those interviewed complained about pressure from steel toe caps. This seemed especially true for workers with bunions, hammertoes, and broad flat feet. The pressure from the steel toe cap produced blisters, corns, and other foot problems.

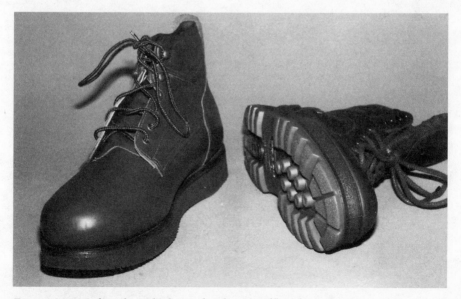

FIGURE 14-2. *Safety shoes: high top, hard toe, waffle sole*

IN A NUTSHELL

In most jobs, there is a chance for foot and ankle injury. The goal is to minimize the risks of injury by adhering to habits and standards of safety in the work place.

Specific areas of occupational injury to the foot include the ankle (ankle fractures), metatarsals and midfoot, toe, and heel. Other injuries relate to sole punctures, burns, and RSD.

To protect the worker against unavoidable injuries, a compensation system is available to provide medical and financial benefits and ensure a safe and healthy work environment. Such a system has been vastly improved with close doctor-employer cooperation, coordination, and commitment to employee welfare. Of course, maintaining a safe work environment is a crucial preventive measure. Safety footwear also contributes to your foot and ankle safety on the job.

CHAPTER 15

Am I Wearing the Right Kind of Shoes?

"To a foot in a shoe, the whole world seems to be paved with leather"
—THE HITOPADESA I, c. 500

INTRODUCTION

Did Cinderella have a problem with her feet from the glass slipper? Most likely! During a recent four-hour shoe symposium at the Academy of Orthopedic Surgeons, Dr. Michael Coughlin reported on all his toe surgeries over the last fifteen years. The surgeries included bunions,

> The shape and size of shoes for your feet are as important as the size of the tires on your car. Whether it is day-to-day walking or demanding sports, comfort and function are the key words. When in doubt, seek the advice of a specialist. It is well worth the investment.

bunionettes, hammertoes, and others. Eighty-five percent of these surgeries were performed on women. Clearly, the shoe is guilty!

Faulty-fitting shoes are the major contributor to many foot problems. High heels and pointed toes are the biggest culprits. Also, there are major inconsistencies in shoe sizes and shapes. There is also a very inadequate selection of shoes with wider, extra depth shoe toe boxes.

In the past, society has dictated fashion over function. An interesting comparison was made between the ancient Chinese custom of binding women's feet and the more recent fashion of spiked high heel shoes. Both examples demonstrate how the woman's foot has been severely restricted and squeezed. The history of the Chinese foot binding technique on foot function and anatomy has been well documented. The average adult female bound foot was only three-and-one-half inches long. The foot ended up deformed, shortened, arthritic, and relatively nonfunctional, requiring a hobbling gate. Wearing narrow, poorly fitting shoes can have less dramatic but still disabling effects.

The fact that over eighty percent of people have two different-sized feet compounds the problem. Many people have a full size difference in

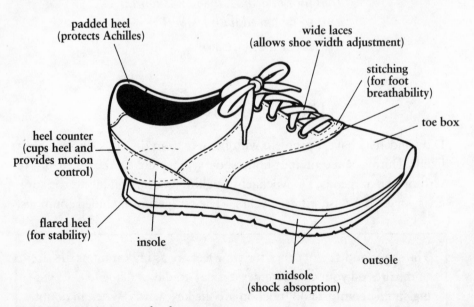

DIAGRAM 15-1 *Anatomy of a shoe*

either width or length between their two feet. Try to find shoes that take this into consideration! One foot gets "stuffed" into a shoe that does not fit properly, even though the shoes may look attractive.

Historically, shoe sizing was developed from the English system dating back to the fourteenth century. Barley corns were used for the unit of measure with three corns equaling one inch. One barley corn equaled one size increase, and thirty-nine barley corns (thirteen inches) was considered the largest foot

Minor adjustments in shoe length were also built into the system for each width increase. But the wider shoe (for example, an 8E versus an 8A) was actually one-third-inch longer, as well. These variations continue to be confusing and are not always subject to quality control.

WHAT SHOULD YOU CONSIDER FOR PROPER SHOE FIT?

There are shoes for a variety of functions like work, casual living, formal dress, and sports. When making shoe selections, it is important to consider the function of the shoe, not just appearance.

There are two key factors to proper shoe fit: Shoe shape and shoe size. Shoe size and matching the size to your foot is no easy task. The correct shoe shape is determined by the shape of your foot. The shape of a shoe is based on a last or form over which the shoe is fabricated. Lasts vary from one manufacturer to another which makes shoe selection and shoe fit difficult. Figure 15-2 illustrates select shoe shapes, including an inflare last, an out-flare last, and a combination last.

Shoe Anatomy

A key component of a shoe is the shank. The shank is the part of the shoe that extends from the heel to the break or flexible toe area. The trick is to fit the shank length to your arch length. Shanks may be flexible, semi-rigid, or rigid.

The curve and flex of the shoe have a lot to do with the shape and configuration of the upper shoe. The shape of the toe box (pointed, rounded, or squared) and its depth are also important considerations. Extra depth, rounded, or squared toe boxes on shoes accommodate difficult-to-fit larger or deformed feet. This type of shoe should be everyone's choice for everyday shoes.

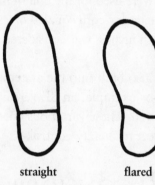

straight   flared   combination narrow   bunion last
                                     heel wide forefoot

DIAGRAM 15-2 *Some type of shoe lasts (shapes)*

DIAGRAM 15-3 *Shoe depth: shallow toe box (top) and extra depth toe box (bottom)*

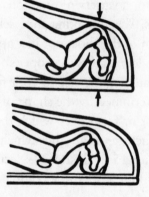

DIAGRAM 15-4 *Shoe shape: wide toe box (left) and pointed and narrow toe box (right)*

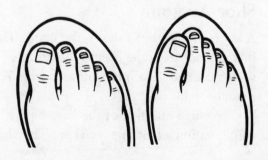

Lace up shoes allow considerable adjustability in shoe fit. This type of shoe should be considered when foot problems exist. The Blucher and Balmoral lace stays are the common patterns. Blucher is considered the best. Some shoe designs vary the position of the eyelets so you can alter your lacing technique for a better grip of your heel. For a narrow heel, form a small loop by threading the lace from the second-to-the-top eyelet to the top hole on each side. Thread the opposite lace through each loop before tying the laces tightly. If your heel is narrow and your forefoot is wide, use two laces. Thread one from the middle to the top forming the loop lace, and tie tightly. Thread the other from the middle to the bottom, lace, and tie loosely.

High heel shoes have very little vamp (the lower part of the upper shoe). As a result, to hold the shoe on the foot properly, the vamp has to fit snugly. Often it fits too snugly which makes it discomforting and sloppy. The high angle of loading on the ball of the foot from this type of shoe puts excessive pressure on the metatarsals. This often leads to metatarsalgia and/or bunions, hammertoes, or other foot problems.

Another major complaint in finding proper shoes that I often hear is, "When I find a shoe comfortable shoe for the front of my foot, my heel slips out." Most shoes are designed so that as the width of the forefoot increases, the width of the heel increases as well. A recent survey of 356 women demonstrated that in many cases, the forefoot width increase was much larger than the heel width.

There is another factor that adds to the shoe fit problem. As the foot matures (ages), the forefoot ligaments tend to loosen and the foot spreads more. This problem is now more recognized and more combination lasts (broad forefoot and narrow heel lasts) are being manufactured. There also is heavier emphasis nowadays in shoe advertising and manufacturing on comfort and function rather than just fashion. But regardless of what you hear or read, do yourself a favor and, like the old saying advises, "If the shoe fits, wear it."

In summary, proper shoe fit requires the following:

• Shape or last design with proper toe depth and shape, proper instep (vamp) depth, proper heel width, and proper curve (flare) of the shoe.

- Proper shoe size including heel to toe length, arch length (heel to widest part of the ball of the foot), and forefoot width (AAA to EEE, and so on).

Keep in mind that high heel shoes increase pressure on the forefoot by at least fifty percent. Consider lower heels and spend less time in high heels. Your feet will be happier!

Suggestions for Shoe Fitting

Here are some suggestions to think about when getting shoes that fit:

- Measure both feet—most of us have mismatched feet.
- Measure feet at least every year. Foot sizes (especially the forefoot) change with aging.
- Measure and fit shoes at the end of the day, as your feet swell from prolonged use.
- ALWAYS stand when measuring feet, as the toes spread while standing.
- Stand on tiptoes and repeat the measurement of the ball of your foot width.
- Fit the shoe you buy to your longer foot. Allow three-eights- to one-half-inch (approximately one finger tip width) clearance for your longest toe.
- Women may consider looking at men's shoes which allow more toe clearance (extra depth). A woman's shoe is usually two sizes smaller than a man's shoe. For example, men's size seven is equal to women's size nine.
- Make sure your heel does not slip out of the shoe during walking. If this is a problem, consider:
    - Lace shoes (Blucher)
    - Shoes with higher backs—t-straps, sling backs, and so forth
    - Combination lasts
    - Pads inside the heel for better fit
    - The advice of a certified pedorthist

- Remember that brand sizes differ. Foreign brands may have less quality control. Also watch for ridges, poor stitching, and other imperfections that can spell trouble for your feet.

- Ensure that the material of the shoe allows your foot to breathe (leather can breathe).

- Outline your foot. While standing, have someone carefully outline your foot on paper. Then compare your foot outline with an outline of your shoes. If the shoe outline is smaller, look out!

  Make a forefoot width card and carry it with you when you purchase shoes. Compare the widest part of the shoe forefoot to your card. The shoe should equal or be no more than 1/4 inch less than your forefoot width. Athletic shoes should be equal in width because the stress is much greater during sports and exercise.

  If the shoes in your closet don't fit the forefoot width card, do your feet a favor and don't wear them. Give them away when you can bear to part with them.

- Socks need to fit as well. Socks that are too long, bunch, or crease can cause pressure. Socks that are too short constrict the toes and can cause deformities. In general, socks should be three-eights-inch longer than your foot.

WHAT ABOUT SPORTS SHOES

Sports shoes are designed specifically for the demands and stresses a particular sport places on the foot. Even the position an athlete plays on a team (running back versus lineman, and so on) can make a difference. Sports shoe manufacturers collect data on specific foot injuries related to a sport, and shoe characteristics are changed to prevent such injuries.

Support and shock absorption cannot be overlooked in sports shoes. Cushioning (shock absorption) is altered by the type or thickness of the sole material of the shoe. By controlling the shoe material's hardness on the inner or outer parts of the midsole, the amount of pronation or supination may be altered. The rigidity of the heel counter and extending it further toward the toes on either the inside or outside of the shoe can aid in motion control.

The amount of flex in a shoe also allows for better foot shock absorption. However, if you have pain across the joint of your toes (MTP joints) or you have sprained your toes, a more rigid toe flex or a rocker sole may be necessary.

Ankle support can be altered by the type of sports shoe you wear. High tops or even higher heel counters can provide better ankle protection. Sports that involve jumping use this design of shoe for that reason.

The type of shoe sole (waffle, cleats, or smooth) surface needs to be considered for specific activities. For example, in tennis, a smooth sole for sliding is desirable, while soccer requires cleats.

Limited space makes it difficult to discuss appropriate shoes for every sport. But these suggestions should be seriously considered. A pedorthist is specifically trained in shoe fitting and supports. He or she should be consulted if you have problems finding shoes. See the PFA (Pedorthic Footwear Association) directory to find a licensed pedorthist in your area.

RUNNING SHOES

In selecting the proper running shoe, there are some basic rules to follow. Much of the shoe industry's "scientific" information is a sales pitch. A safe rule to follow is if you have found comfortable running shoes, continue to use them. However, do not continue to wear these shoes beyond their natural life expectancy by using shoe glue, etc. All shoe materials tend to bottom out or change with use. Adding non-conforming materials alters the basic shoe.

You should analyze your own foot structure before buying running shoes. For example, is your arch high and are your ligaments tight? Are there any calluses on your feet that indicate areas of high pressure? The location of these calluses should be identified. If there are calluses on the bottom of your foot toward the small toe, it suggests that you have a supination stress pattern. Conversely, if you have a pancake arch or calluses on the inside arch and big toe area, or if your heel is angled outward (everted), you have a pronation stress pattern.

A history of shin splints also suggests a pronation problem. In most cases, a supinated or high arched foot requires a more shock absorbing type of shoe. A flat or pronating foot should have a more supportive type of shoe.

The pattern of sole wear often helps determine the type of foot anatomy you have. Limited heel wear suggests a midfoot striker which is often associated with excess stress on the Achilles tendon (tendinitis). Excessive outside heel wear that extends to the lateral midsole suggests an excess supination problem. A medial (inside) broken down heel counter is a tipoff that you are pronating excessively.

There are numerous brands of running shoes available. There are also many running books and magazine articles that rate running shoes for consumers. The shoe fitting suggestions in this chapter are important to consider when choosing a running shoe. The cost of the shoe does not mean it is better. It is the quality of stitching, a padded and supportive heel counter, and breathable material that you should examine. Adequate toe flex with no pressure applied to any one area is important. Alternating eyelets and an extra eyelet at the ankle area allows for better control of heel fit. Running shoes lose their natural durability after running 250 to 300 miles. They should be replaced at about that time.

When ankle instability (giving way, ankle sprains) is a problem, the more outflared sole provides additional support to the ankle. Certain shoes have more outflare than others. Hyperpronation controls vary from company to company. Variable midsole materials with harder medial heel and arch material, slight tilting of the heel of the shoe inward

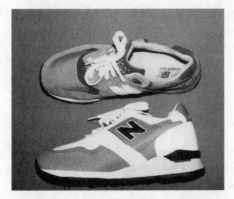

FIGURE 15-5. *Running shoe with flared heel and firm counter motion control*

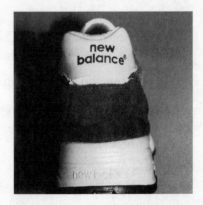

FIGURE 15-6. *Running shoe with flared heel*

(medial heel wedge), or extended medial counters are examples. If you are a pronator, too much outflare only exaggerates your problem.

It is worth noting that running and jogging shoes make very good walking shoes. They can be used as everyday shoes as well.

SHOE MODIFICATIONS INSIDE AND OUTSIDE THE SHOE

Certain foot problems like bunions, metatarsalgia, and arthritis still cause feet to hurt, despite properly fitting shoes. Simple adjustments by a pedorthist can be of great help. Simple shoe stretching can relieve the pressure point of bunions, hammertoes, or bunionettes. A small slit in the toe box or replacing a section of the toe box with a more elastic type of material can bring a lot of comfort. Open toe sandals or strap-on modified cast shoes may accommodate swelling and deformity. They are especially useful in the post-operative or injury recovery period.

There are a number of shoe adjustments that address shoe problems. These modifications should be done by a skilled shoe repair person or a pedorthist:

- **Heel and sole lifts**—used in adjusting short leg problems.

- **Heel cushion**—used in arthritis conditions.

- **Rocker sole and steel shank**—helpful for arthritis of the toes or feet.

- **Metatarsal bars**—have the same function as rocker soles and are used for metatarsalgia. The pressure is transferred toward the heel and away from the ball of the foot.

- **High top shoes with straps**—provide ankle stability.

- **Heel wedges or sole wedges**—used in changing the angle of pressures on the foot, ankle, or knee. They may be used with knee arthritis as well.

- **Heel flares**—used with progressing flat foot (pronation) on the inside heel or on the outside of the heel if the ankle is unstable (supination).

- **Medial (inside) or lateral (outside) stabilizer**—extension of the heel counter to include inside (pronation) or outside (supination) problems.

- **Thermo-molded shoe**—new shoes whose shape can be easily changed by heating and stretching. They are used with a significant deformity resulting from diabetes or rheumatoid arthritis. Cushioned inserts (plastazote) that mold to the foot with walking are part of these special shoes.

- **Custom shoes**—necessary for severe deformities and are made from a cast of the foot.

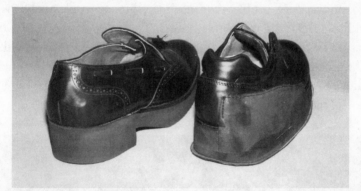

FIGURE 15-7A. *Shoe modifications: Left shows elevated heel and sole for short leg, rocker sole to relieve pressure on ankle and ball of foot. Right shows lateral stabilizer to help prevent excessive supination and unstable ankles.*

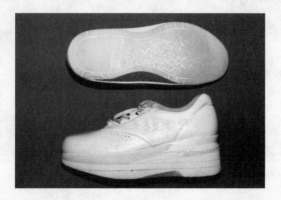

FIGURE 15-7B. *Types of orthotics over-the-counter and custom made.*

Many shoe adjustments have the advantage of being less expensive and can be completed quickly. One of their limitations is a lack of flexibility (the adjustment is confined to one pair of shoes). Also, some shoes cannot be adjusted. So inserts play an important role in foot problems.

ORTHOTICS AND INTERNAL PADS

Orthotics are molded inserts or standard inserts placed inside the shoe. The purpose is to relieve pressures and/or help control abnormal motion like supination or pronation. Simple self-applied pads or over-the-counter inserts are usually tried first because of the cost savings. Unfortunately, some common foot problems (even knee, hip, or back problems) only respond to specialized molded supports. These are made from a cast or impression of the foot. The problem is they do take up space within the shoe. Many unhappy patients have been issued supports only to find that they don't fit in any of these shoes. To gain the extra space, the liner in the shoe is removed and replaced with the orthotic.

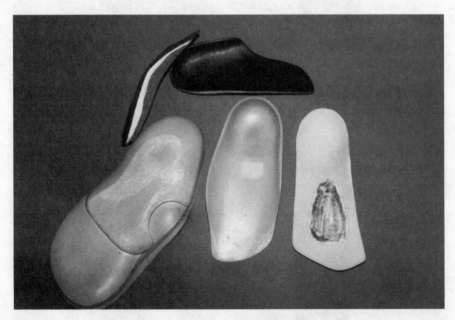

FIGURE 15-8. *Types of orthotics over-the-counter and custom made*

SHOE INSERT DEVICES

There are several shoe devices worth considering:

- **Spenko**—over the counter cushion arch support.
- **Dr. Scholl's pads**—very good shock absorbers.
- **Metatarsal pads**—stick-in-shoe type of simple pad which may relieve metatarsalgia or callus pain.
- **Flexible accommodative orthotics**—made from a mold of the foot. Relieves the diabetic foot or a tight foot.
- **Semi-rigid orthotics**—help control abnormal foot motion and provide some shock absorption. For recurrent shin splints, flexible foot with pronation problems, knee cap problems.
- **Rigid orthotics**—for motion control for flexible foot deformity but not shock absorbing. Orthotic fabrication is still an inexact science. Orthotics only fit certain shoes and are expensive. They frequently require adjustments and should not be prescribed until less expensive devices have been tried.

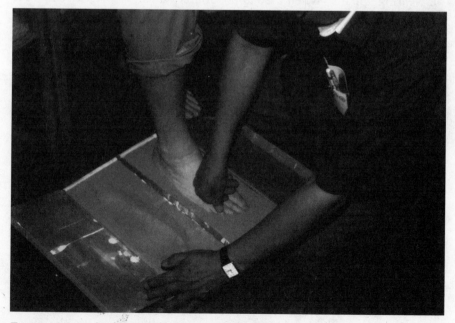

FIGURE 15-9 *Making the mold for custom orthotics*

A common mistake is to wear the new orthotic or foot altering device for too long without allowing the foot adequate time to adjust. You should start by wearing the device for one or two hours a day and increase the time gradually. Try them for everyday activities before wearing them for your sport.

BRACES

Sometimes, additional support is necessary in order to get stability and function in certain ankle and foot problems. Two basic designs for braces exist: a metal upright brace that inserts into the shoe sole, or a plastic AFO (ankle-foot orthosis) that fits into the shoe and extends up the back of the calf. The AFO is lighter and less noticeable, but is not tolerated by people whose legs tend to swell or change size.

There are sometimes shoe fitting problems using this brace, as well. The external bar brace is stronger and accommodates swelling. By altering the hinge spring mechanism at the ankle, it can also assist in lifting the toes in patients with leg weakness or neuropathy. A brace should be regarded as a helpful device and should be considered just another piece of wearing apparel. When used appropriately, it can sometimes eliminate the need for surgery. Braces are used commonly:

- After a stroke.
- By diabetics with deformed/unstable foot or ankle problems.
- For nerve injuries.
- For painful arthritis when limiting painful motion is the goal. It is a substitute for a cast or fusion surgery.

The guidance and advice of an orthotist (brace specialist) is important because the brace needs to have the proper fit and be made of the appropriate material in order to accomplish its purpose.

IN A NUTSHELL

The shape of your feet should determine the shape of the shoes you buy. Your feet may be different sizes and need enough width, depth, and length to be IMMEDIATELY comfortable.

Orthotics and shoe devices like metatarsal pads can help relieve many foot problems, but they need enough room in your shoes to do the right job.

There are shoes specially designed for specific sports, based on studies of common sports injuries and stresses that are natural to that sport. Be sure the shoes you wear for the sport are appropriate, comfortable, and not worn out.

DOCTOR'S CORNER: QUESTIONS AND ANSWERS

I used to wear orthopedic shoes for my bunions. Where can I find these shoes now?

Shoe companies now make a wide variety of walking shoes that do the same thing as "orthopedic" shoes did after World War II. The key words here are the extra depth flexibility and shock absorbing ability that these shoes provide to accommodate your bunions. Many shoe stores have licensed pedorthists to help you with your shoe selection and fit.

What kind of running shoe should I buy?

There are so many running shoes on the market now that the selection is confusing. These shoes are designed to do specific things, but the important things to consider are *your* specific feet! If you supinate or pronate when you run, the distances and speed you run and the surface you run on are some of the things that must be considered. You may need an evaluation by a sports medicine specialist to determine the best shoe for your feet.

Price is not the best judge of a good shoe and shoe manufacturing is not an exact science either. If you have found comfortable functional running shoes, keep using them. Make sure that you replace them when they are worn out.

I have some expensive sandals that I like. Is it harmful for my feet to wear them?

There are some good sandals on today's market that provide better shock absorption and support than in the past. If yours are comfortable, by all means wear them. I would suggest good walking shoes for long distances, however.

TERMS TO REMEMBER

Flare: Curve of a shoe.

Flexible accommodative orthotics: Orthotics made from a mold of the foot. It is used to relieve the diabetic foot or a tight foot.

Heel and sole lift: A device used in adjusting short leg problems.

Heel cushion: A cushion used in arthritis conditions.

Heel flares: Used with progressing flat foot (pronation) or on the outside of the heel if the ankle is unstable (supination).

Heel/sole wedge: Used to change the angle of pressures on the foot, ankle, or knee.

High-top shoes with straps: Shoes with a unique function of providing ankle stability.

Last: The form over which a shoe is constructed.

Lateral stabilizer: Extension of the heel counter to include outside (supination) problems.

Medial stabilizer: Extension of the heel counter to include inside (pronation) problems.

Metatarsal bar: Similar to a rocker sole. It is used for metatarsalgia. The pressure is transferred toward the heel and away from the ball of the foot.

Metatarsal pad: Stick-in-shoe type of simple pad which may relieve metatarsalgia or callus pain.

Orthotics: Molded or standard inserts which are placed inside the shoe.

Pedorthist: A specialist in shoe inserts (orthotics).

Rigid orthotics: Special orthotics used for motion control for flexible foot deformity but not shock absorbing.

Rocker sole: A sole that helps the arthritis of the toes or foot.

Semi-rigid orthotics: Special orthotics that help control abnormal foot motion and provide some shock absorption.

Shank: The part of a shoe that extends from the heel to the break or flexible toe area.

Spenko: Over-the-counter cushion arch support.

Thermo-molded shoe: Custom shoe made from the mold of the foot.

Toe box: The front of the shoe (rounded or pointed) that houses toes.

Vamp: The lower part of the upper shoe.

CHAPTER 16

Physical Therapy and Rehabilitation

INTRODUCTION

In the preceding chapters, we discussed basic foot problems and medical and surgical treatments. An important component in the whole process is rehabilitation. It is a critical step, in that the goal of rehabilitation is to return a person to maximum function. In contrast, the purpose of physical therapy is to decrease swelling, increase Range Of Motion (ROM),

Physical therapy helps you begin your rehabilitation after surgery, an injury, or other problems through exercises, modalities, and instruction. The goals of this physical therapy are to help recover range of motion, reduce swelling, learn exercise techniques, and prevent injury.

and improve the patient's coordination, strength, and endurance. A high percentage of people with foot and ankle injuries will have a reinjury. Many of these problems result from incomplete rehabilitation of their original injury. Others stem from a failure to correct their sports training and obtain appropriate instruction in running, throwing, and other sports techniques. This is why physical therapy has become an integral part of foot and ankle injury treatment.

One of the key players in rehabilitation is the physical therapist. These are medical professionals specifically trained to assist in meeting these goals. The patient's present condition and recreational and occupational aims are carefully evaluated. Overall, aerobic fitness also needs to be checked. Although the most important component of physical therapy is *exercise*, there are other forms of therapy such as massage, heat, and other modalities best used when combined with an exercise program.

A general physical therapy assessment looks at swelling, loss of ROM and strength, tenderness (pain location), instability (balance), and endurance. Any deficiency in these areas can lead to pain and a loss of function. So all these factors must be treated to ensure proper healing. All exercises included in this chapter address each particular foot and ankle problem accordingly.

Keep in mind that physical exercise serves a number of purposes such as recovering lost motion resulting from surgery or cast immobilization, returning muscles to their normal tone, and regaining or improving balance skills. These are goals that are usually attained in stages and as quickly after surgery or injury as the situation warrants. In this chapter, we focus on physical therapy, the various approaches used by physical therapists, and taping techniques. We also talk about self-treatment, preventing reinjuries, and incorporating proper training such as warmups and cooldowns into your exercise plan.

THE REHABILITATION PROCESS

Rehabilitation is viewed as a three-step process: The acute swelling inflammatory phase, the intermediate phase, and the full return to activity phase. The process also focuses on certain noninjury foot problems such as arthritis, with its residual stiffness, chronic swelling, instability problems of the ankle or foot, and acute and chronic (long lasting) ligament and tendon (tendinitis) problems. Rehabilitation means muscle retraining, coordination drills, and specific muscle strengthening and muscle balancing exercises.

In rehabilitation, the focus is on the proper technique, since choice of the wrong technique could easily work against you. So training is designed around the specific tasks or sports movements the patient actually performs. The "normal" opposite leg and foot are included in the exercise program to avoid creating a muscle imbalance. The goal of physical therapy is to design a program fitted to the patient's specific needs and environment that eventually will be performed in one's own home. Once implemented, the exercise program should continue indefinitely.

Acute Injury Treatment

An acute injury requires starting treatment as soon as possible. After a foot or ankle injury, for example, it is critical to control swelling. Swelling is the way your body protects itself from further trauma. It is also the tissue's response to the trauma. Immediately after an injury, the best treatment is to use RICE as explained below. You'll recognize this discussion from chapter 12.

Rest. Physical therapists commonly observe patients mistakenly trying to "limp their way through an injury under the 'no pain no gain' concept." Frequent complaints of hip, knee, or back pain, in addition to pain stemming from the injury, are the result of "limping." Crutches, a walker, or a cane to assist ambulation in the early stages of the injury is a better solution. These devices help you walk "normally," while you are able to take some weight off the injured foot or leg. They also serve to decrease stress to the tissues and allow you to maintain a normal gait pattern.

Ice. For proper use of ice, refer to the physical therapy modalities section in this chapter.

Compression. Using an Ace wrap can decrease swelling. A *word to the wise* is not to wear these bandages at night because of possible circulation difficulties. When you wrap, start at your toes and work up the leg. Take care not to wrap the area too tightly, which could restrict circulation. If you feel numbness or tingling, increased swelling in the toes, or more pain, you must loosen or remove the wrap immediately.

Elevation. An important step is to keep your leg above the level of your heart to help decrease swelling of your foot or ankle. This should assist the venous return of the blood to your heart.

Exercises for Ankle Sprains and Soft Tissue Injuries

For most ankle sprains and soft tissue injuries, total immobilization (casting) has been replaced by early, safe motion exercises. These exercises allow the leg muscle pumping action to decrease swelling and to regain range of motion. There are several early stage exercises to choose from. Each exercise has a special purpose and provides unique benefits.

Early Stage Exercises

- **Ankle pumps.** Moving the ankle up and down in a pumping motion is crucial to decreasing swelling, especially when you are sitting. This exercise is used with almost all acute soft tissue injuries, including sprains.
- **Towel stretches.** Place a towel around the ball of the foot and hold both ends in your hands. Relax the muscles in your lower leg and pull the towel slowly toward you until you feel a mild tension in your calf; then hold for thirty seconds. Try to relax. It is impor-

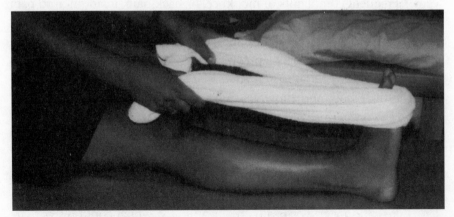

FIGURE 16-1. *Towel stretch*

tant to perform this prestretch before you even get out of bed. It will relieve early morning pain. Repeat this stretch three times and try to do it three or four times a day. See figure 16-1.

- **Retrograde massage.** The focus of this exercise is to reduce swelling. The injured area is massaged with motion toward the direction of the heart. It is not unusual to find the exercise painful right after the injury.

- **Alphabet exercises.** The idea behind this exercise is to try to "write out" the alphabet in the air with your ankle. This simulates ankle motion in all directions. It is an excellent technique to help gain and maintain motion in all joints of the foot. It is also a good exercise to keep your mind off the injury and is usually recommended later in acute soft tissue injuries, when pain and swelling have subsided.

- **Toe Towel Curls.** Crunching up a towel with your toes or picking up marbles with your toes helps decrease swelling in the forefoot. It can be a challenging exercise.

- **Ankle circles.** This exercise is used to maintain ankle and foot motion. Ankle circles are a three-step process. First, the foot is turned slowly in a circle clockwise. Then, the motion is repeated counter-clockwise. Third, the circles are gradually increased in size as pain and swelling permit. The exercise is not normally recommended in the early recovery period after sprains.

- **Ankle Isometrics.** Isometric exercises are designed to strengthen or help maintain muscle strength by contracting the muscle *without* moving any joint. They should be painless, or nearly so, and are used early and throughout the rehabilitation program. As described, this exercise applies to the right ankle, so reverse the procedure for the left.

  - Cross your left foot over and on top of your right foot. Pull up with your right foot and push down with your left. Hold for six seconds and relax. Repeat a prescribed set of times.

  - Cross your left foot under your right foot, then push down with the right foot and up with the left.

- Place your feet so both big toes are facing each other. Press inward with both feet.
- Place your feet so both little toes are next to each other. Push outward with both feet.

COMMONLY USED PHYSICAL THERAPY TREATMENTS

Cold Versus Heat Treatment

Ice. Ice is used to reduce blood flow to the injured area and to control and reduce swelling for the first several weeks while swelling from the injury persists. Ice is applied for fifteen to twenty minutes, followed by four or five minutes off. A light towel or pillowcase should be applied between the skin and the ice. A great trick of the trade that physical therapists use is applying a bag of frozen peas or corn to the injured area instead of ice. Frozen vegetables in plastic bags mold to the joints well and can be refrozen (but don't eat the product).

Icing for more than twenty minutes at a time is not good because the blood vessels in the skin dilate, which increases blood flow and swelling. This is the very cycle you should avoid.

Ice massage has been known to help decrease swelling. One way is to freeze water in a dixie cup, then remove the paper, and rub the ice around the injured area for six to eight minutes. You should apply ice massage for a shorter time because it cools the area faster than icing.

Another ice technique is a cryopump. The pump is ice-cooled and then strapped on the injured foot or leg. It is intermittently inflated and deflated to simulate the normal pumping action of the leg or foot muscles. This is an effective technique, although cost is a factor. You'll find a cryopump commonly used by athletes whose rapid recovery is critical.

Heat. As you probably know, heat increases blood flow to the injured area, which makes swelling worse. Because of this, it is not recommended for at least several weeks after injury. There are several heat variations:

- **Dry heat.** A heating pad is applied directly to the skin for twenty minutes at a time. It helps increase blood flow and improve ROM.

- **Moist heat.** Moist heat increases flexibility of your muscles. It is occasionally used to increase motion after the acute phase of the injury has stabilized. A warm towel, warm bath, or moist heating pad are the choices available.

- **Contrast bath.** This type of bath alternates heat and cold, with the heat, increasing circulation and blood flow and the cold decreasing swelling. It is used in the later period of acute injury when mild swelling and stiffness persist but the initial injury symptoms and severe swelling have abated. The procedure is as follows:

  - Use cold water (50 to 65 degrees Fahrenheit) for one minute.

  - Use hot water (100 to 110 degrees Fahrenheit) for three to five minutes.

  - Alternate these baths four to five times, always ending in cold water to limit swelling.

Ultrasound

This form of deep heating from sound waves is used by physical therapists to increase tissue temperature and improve circulation. Many imitation products are on the market, but fail to perform the same function. By using ultrasound over an inflammation area secondary to muscle tightness, we are attempting to achieve two goals: increasing tissue temperature to improve flexibility and promoting circulation to decrease swelling.

Another method of ultrasound is called phonophoresis. This uses an ultrasound current and a prescription topical anti-inflammatory (hydrocortisone) to allow the medication to penetrate into the tissue and reduce inflammation.

A third method to reduce inflammation is Ionotophoresis. This method uses a low grade direct current over a pad saturated with an anti-inflammatory medication that is driven into the inflamed tissue. Improved results are commonly seen after as few as three treatments.

Electric stimulation covers a variety of machines, frequencies, and functions. For example, the Interferrential is a machine that produces a micromassage effect which helps reduce swelling. Vibrational signals also help decrease pain.

Stretching

Patients often ask, "Why do my physical therapist and doctor recommend stretching my injured part?" Well, take tendinitis or torn tendons. These injuries heal by scar tissue which contracts or shortens over time as healing occurs. When this happens, it causes loss of flexibility and increases the chance of reinjury when the patient resumes activity. The stretching helps prevent that and should be done gently and only *gradually* increased. The tendons and ligaments are protected with controlled motion and rest.

The recommendations are to stretch until creating a gentle tension and holding it for thirty seconds. The stretch should be slow and static—no bouncing. This should be repeated three to five times. The more stretching you do, the better off you will be. Actually, stretching should be included in your daily exercise and daily life. Before you get out of bed, you should do a specific calf and foot prestretch routine if you have heel pain or plantar fasciitiis. The cooldown is as important as the warmup and will help prevent muscle soreness and cramping at the end of the exercise. Therefore, stretching after exercise should not be overlooked.

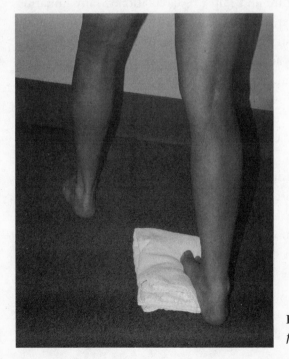

FIGURE 16-2. *Stretch heel cord-forefoot locked*

Most people try to stretch their calf muscles by leaning forward against a wall. However, many physical therapists feel that this stretch is ineffective without modification. Since most of us have an inadequate arch, the arch should be firmly supported, especially if you are stretching barefoot or in an unsupported shoe. One way of modifying the traditional stretch is to place a one-inch towel roll on the inside half (from the big toe to the second toe) of your foot and heel. Now you can do the stretching shown in figure 16-2.

Proper stretching is done in three phases:

- With the leg you're stretching placed behind your other leg, keep your back knee straight and both heels firmly on the floor.
- Lean into the wall by bending your front knee forward. You should feel a constant stretch in your calf, but no pain.
- When this becomes easy, increase your distance from the wall.

To stretch the soleus (part of your calf muscle), you perform the same stretch, except you bend both knees and you do not lean as aggressively into the wall. A stretch should be felt lower in the Achilles tendon region. None of these stretches should produce pain. If you have pain, you are doing the stretches too aggressively.

Stretching the Plantar Fascia

The plantar fascia is probably the easiest part of your foot/ankle to stretch and is the least felt. There are two methods to stretch it: sitting and standing. The *sitting* exercise involves pulling your toes up toward the direction of your head from the ball of your foot. It is easy to feel with your hands how tight the fascia is on the inside of your arch. The *standing* exercise involves placing the ball of your foot on the floor and leaning forward on your toes. This lifts the heel and transfers the weight forward, while it keeps the ball of the foot on the floor. The plantar and heel cord prestretch routine for those with heel pain or fasciitis is *extremely important*. It is most painful to do first thing in the morning, but this stretch is very beneficial and worth your time and effort.

Whether sitting or standing, to relieve pain in the plantar fascia some people find rolling their foot over a ball (like a tennis ball) helps. Massaging your foot can also help reduce pain.

Strengthening Exercises

Before talking about strengthening exercises, keep in mind the four motions of the ankle joint:

- **Plantar flexion**—moving the toes down to the floor.
- **Dorsi flexion**—moving the toes up.
- **Inversion**—bringing the big toe toward the midline.
- **Eversion**—moving the foot away from the midline.

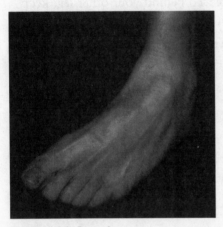

FIGURE 16-3. *Inversion*

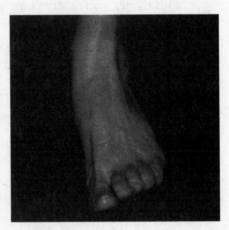

FIGURE 16-4. *Eversion*

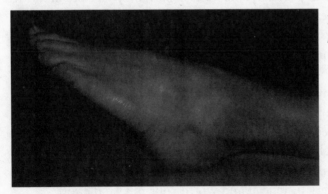

FIGURE 16-5. *Plantar flexion*

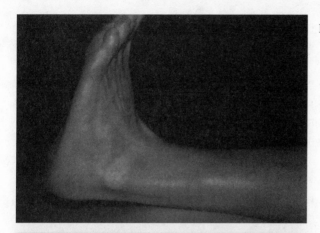

FIGURE 16-6. *Dorsiflexion*

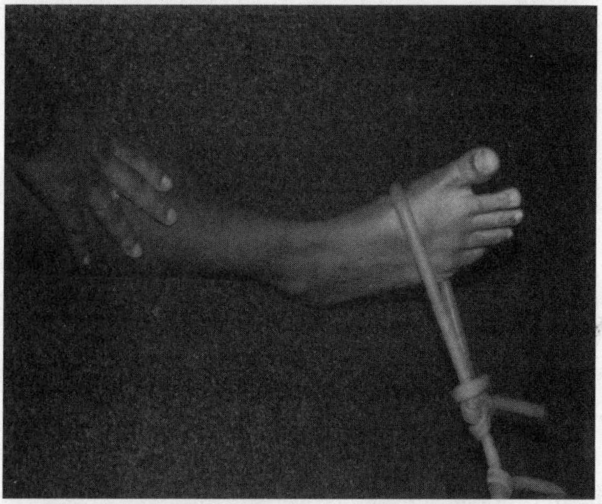

FIGURE 16-7. *Rubber tubing exercise*

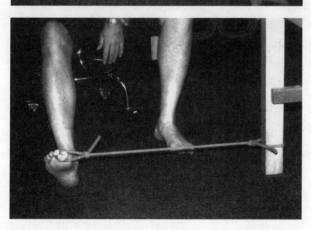

FIGURE 16-8. *Rubber tubing exercises using a table leg*

It is imperative to strengthen the muscles that control these motions after an injury. The muscles that control plantar flexion are in the back of your calf. They are a very strong muscle group which can be built up by using resistive bands and calf raises. One common strengthening exercise uses rubber tubing. A piece of rubber tubing two to three feet long and one-quarter inch in diameter is used to perform the exercise. The procedure is simple. Sit with your legs out straight and place the tube around your toes. Hold the ends in your hands and push your foot down against the band.

Another rubber tubing exercise starts with fastening the tubing around the leg of a bed or other heavy piece of furniture. For the resistive eversion exercise, place the foot into the rubber tubing and twist your ankle in the direction of your little toe.

The peroneal muscles or ankle evertors are the primary ankle stabilizers. To best strengthen this group of muscles, point your toes toward the floor and push the outside of your foot outward. A rubber tubing for dynamic strengthening or a stable object like a desk may be used to provide resistance against the active push.

Taping Techniques

Taping is a mechanism used for the treatment, rehabilitation, and prevention of injuries. The major benefit of taping is to support the joints or foot, ankle, and toe ligaments. Taping an injured area is recommended by physicians and physical therapists.

Taping the Plantar Fascia. Low dye taping is especially helpful to runners or people with plantar fasciitis. Tape is applied to the bottom and sides of the foot, using one roll of one-inch tape, one roll of two-inch tape, and moleskin. The procedure is simple:

- Apply the moleskin at the ball of the foot, pulling toward the heel and attaching it to the heel.

- Push the big toe (plantar) down and other toes slightly upward. Apply two or three one-inch strips as described.

- Cover the foot with two-inch strips from the outside to the inside of the foot. See figure 16-9.

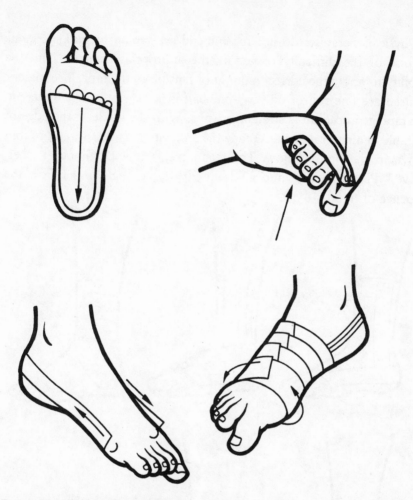

FIGURE 16-9. *Taping plantar fascia*

Ankle Taping. There have been many studies done on the effectiveness of taping versus bracing after rehabilitation from a sprained ankle. A recent study at U.C.L.A. concluded that high top sneakers and a lace-up brace like a Swedo helped to decrease the incidence of recurring ankle sprains. Tape is very supportive for the first twenty minutes of play, but with motion and perspiration, the strength of the tape decreases. Unless it can be freshly applied every twenty minutes, it loses some of its effectiveness in preventing or protecting ankle or foot sprains.

Physical therapists do not recommend self-taping for ankle sprains because of the difficulty of getting the appropriate position and the inability to apply the correct amount of tension to the tape. The materials used are one roll of one-and-one-half-inch tape and tape adherent. The taping procedure is straightforward. With the ankle at the edge of the table in a neutral position, tape the ankle in a manner similar to that shown in the figure below. The technique is called "Gibney basket-weave." Place the foot and ankle at 90 degree angle and follow the sequence of figure 16-10.

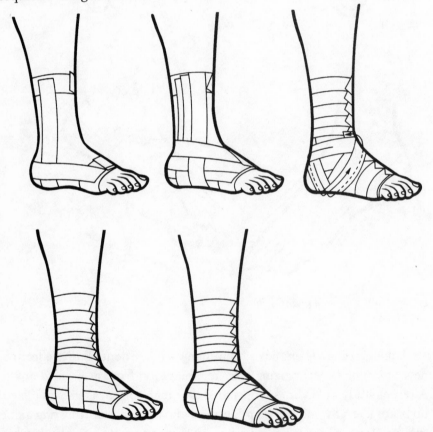

FIGURE 16-10. *Ankle taping*

Turf Toe or Sprained Toe Taping. The purpose of this taping procedure is to limit the range of motion of the "turf toe" or sprained big toe. The materials used are one roll of one-inch tape and tape adherant. Follow the technique as shown in figure 16-11.

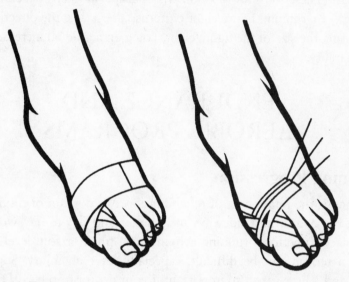

FIGURE 16-11. *Toe taping*

Proprioception-balance

During the past few years, several studies have shown that after a severe ankle sprain, many patients have trouble keeping their balance, especially when they walk on unstable surfaces like grass or sand. Balance-proprioception is your ability to know where your foot is in space. You can test your balance by standing on one foot and counting how long you can maintain an upright position. Your injured leg is then tested the same way.

To work on increasing proprioception, physical therapists recommend standing on your injured leg while doing normal day-to-day activities (brushing your teeth, and so on) When you are able to stand on one leg for 30 seconds and not fall over, try closing your eyes while standing on one foot. Vision plays a major role in balance, and when vision is removed, the proprioceptors in your ankles have to work harder.

A mini-trampoline is used to increase balance by weight shifting, high marching, and jumping. An ankle injury can limit your ability to perform lateral and diagonal patterns in sports. Therapists recommend starting with cuts in a side-to-side motion and then progressing to foot over foot cariocas. (These steps are also known as grapevine steps which improve balance.) By running figure eight patterns, alternating the direction, and decreasing the size of the figure eight, you gain a gradual increase in cutting stability.

ENDURANCE AND AEROBIC PROGRAMS

Running Progression

Running is the final phase of rehabilitation. We do a lot of running forward, backward, and sideways in athletics and day-to-day work. The best place to perform running activities is a track or soft, level surface. Uneven terrain can be difficult, especially after an injury. Supportive shoes and a brace are also important if your doctor or physical therapist recommends them.

Here is a running program that can be modified to suit your specific activity level:

- Jog forward
- Run forward
- Jog backwards (backpedal)
- Run backwards
- Make large figure eights
- Make small figure eights
- Run forward and cut 45 degrees
- Run forward and cut 90 degrees
- Perform obstacle courses
- Do stop/starts

If you are unable to successfully complete all the exercises, you may have to try a more sports-related activity. Good luck!

Beginning a Running Program

Before you start a running program, be sure to consult your doctor for medical clearance. Like any other sport, you must use the proper equipment. Well-fitting, supportive running shoes that are maintained and replaced when they are worn out can save you all kinds of problems and prevent unnecessary injuries.

First, begin jogging on a level surface. Use a track or treadmill only to the point of mild fatigue. Don't be a hero, trying to run a marathon or sprint the pace. Most experts suggest increasing your total running distance by about ten percent a week, and not more than ten percent of the total distance should be on hills. The goal is to move gradually from a controlled distance and environment to an exercise regime that can be performed anytime, anywhere—and this takes time to accomplish.

Remember, there is no such thing as a safe running program that applies to everyone. Some people may want to try a new sport; others want to run because they want to control medical problems.

When Running Hurts

Your body will give you warning signs through pain, muscle aches, and the like. Each running injury is unique and needs special attention or treatment. Figure 16-12 summarizes the warning signs and "what to do" when

Mild Injuries	What to Do
Slight pain at start and pain may reappear.	Increase warm up. Decrease distance and/or incline.

Moderate Injuries	What to do
Moderate pain at start and increase during the run.	Limit or stop running. Bike or swim instead for a few weeks. See your doctor if pain continues.

Severe Injuries	What to do
Loss of motion, stiffness, significant pain that doesn't stop with rest.	Stop running and see your doctor.

FIGURE 16-12. *What to do when running hurts*

running hurts. In any case, if you feel dizzy, have chest pain or tightness, or experience swelling, numbness, or other unusual symptoms while running, simply stop running and check with your doctor right away.

Other Aerobic Programs

Like many people, you might not like to run and your joints might not tolerate the high impact stress that it causes. But you still want an aerobic exercise regimen. Brisk walking using light one- or two-pound weights on your wrists is an excellent exercise. Be sure you do stretching warm-up and cooldown. Start on level surfaces and build up to hills. Proper shoes are very important, as well.

Swimming, water aerobic programs, and biking, either moving or stationary, are all low impact, excellent aerobic and endurance forms of exercise. Find the exercise program that suits your interests, body, and lifestyle best and make it an important part of your life.

IN A NUTSHELL

In this chapter, we have focused on rehabilitation as a set of exercises designed to bring you to maximum function. In terms of acute injury, the best immediate treatment is RICE. For most ankle sprains and soft tissue injuries, early-stage exercises such as ankle pumps, towel stretches, and retrograde massage are available.

The commonly used physical therapy techniques include cold versus heat treatment, ultrasound, and stretching exercises. Each exercise requires knowledge of procedure and discipline.

Taping is often used for the treatment, rehabilitation, and prevention of injuries. Various methods and approaches to taping are included to alert you to the importance of proper taping techniques. If unsure, go to your physical therapist or a specialist to do the job right.

Finally, a running program as an exercise should be designed with you and the type of injury in mind. All running programs must start easy, following a definite procedure, and maintaining a healthy attitude toward the whole process. When you do so, you are investing in a long-term commitment to an injury-free lifestyle.

TERMS TO REMEMBER

Alphabet exercise: An exercise in which the sufferer "writes out" the alphabet in the air with his/her ankle to simulate ankle motion in all directions.

Ankle circles: An exercise to maintain ankle and foot motion; turning the foot slowly clockwise, then counterclockwise and gradually increasing the size of the circles as pain and swelling permit.

Ankle pump: Moving the ankle back and forth in a pumping motion; an exercise used with acute soft tissue injuries, including sprains.

Cryopump: A physical therapy device featuring an intermittent inflating pump that uses cold and compression to reduce swelling.

Dorsi flexion: Moving the toes up—a motion to the ankle joint.

Eversion: Moving the foot away from the midline.

Inversion: Bringing the big toe toward the midline.

Plantar flexion: Moving the toes down to the floor—a motion to the ankle joint.

Rehabilitation: A set of exercises or routines designed to return a person to maximum function.

Retrograde massage: Massaging an injured area with motion toward the direction of the heart to reduce swelling.

Toe towel curls: Crunching up a towel or picking up marbles with the toes to help decrease swelling in the forefoot.

—— ∿ ——

CHAPTER 17

What Do I Need to Know Before Having Surgery and Anesthesia?

INTRODUCTION

In each preceding chapter, we talked about specific foot problems and deformities and how they can be corrected through self-help, medical treatment, or surgical procedures. You should know by now that self-help and medical treatments have limitations. Sometimes, your condition may require surgery. Surgical expectations have also been covered briefly.

Anesthesia is a critical aspect of surgery and deciding whether or not to have surgery is a serious matter. This means you should know about all its aspects, procedures, benefits, and risks. Know your doctor and anesthesiologist before agreeing to elective surgery.

In this chapter, the focus is on standard surgical preparations that you should know about prior to elective foot surgery.

Why devote a separate chapter to foot surgery? Well, every patient I know gets a little nervous a day or so before the "big show." Many patients don't know what surgery entails, what to expect for the intended surgery, or what plan the surgeon will use. Any time there is *elective* foot surgery, it means you the patient have the right to know the plan, the expectations, and answers to all the questions you have in mind *before* surgery is scheduled. There is no such thing as a stupid question when it comes to a vital part of your body. You should know the expected results, possible complications, and the post-op care that you will receive. Since you're the one to decide on the surgery, you should be satisfied with the decision.

PRE-OP ROUTINE

As a routine, part of the pre-op requirements is a medical assessment of your readiness to undergo surgery. This means a chest x-ray, cardiogram, and blood tests which are done the week before scheduled surgery. How extensive the workup has a lot to do with your age, your general health, how recently you had a complete physical, the magnitude of the intended surgery, and the type of anesthesia to be administered. During this time, you will also meet with the anesthesiologist as part of the planning phase of the surgery. The anesthesiologist is a physician trained in administering and handling all forms of anesthesia and its complications.

Most foot surgery is done on an out-patient basis. A few days before surgery, you will meet with the day surgery nurse who handles lab studies that were not done during your medical evaluation. Day surgery personnel will brief you about the recovery room and how long you most likely will stay in observation. See figure 17-1 for a general flowchart of pre-op procedure.

The evening before surgery, you are usually given a medication to help you relax. You will be instructed not to eat or drink any liquids after midnight. If you develop a cold or cough anytime before surgery, your doctor should be notified immediately. You should also plan on having a responsible adult stay with you and drive you home after surgery.

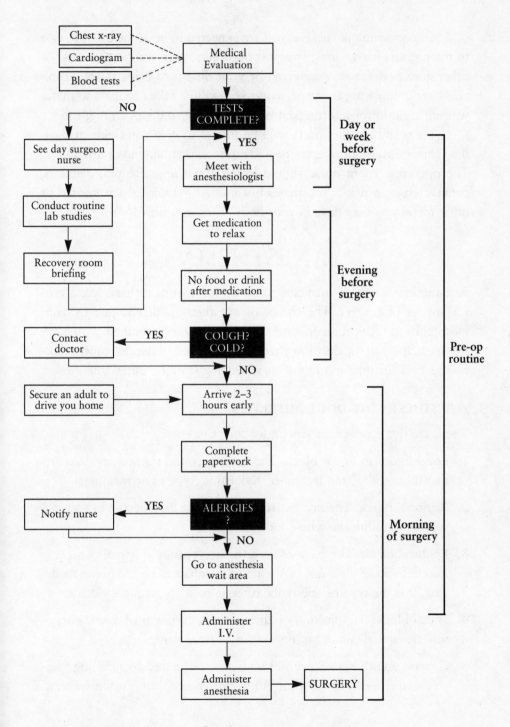

FIGURE 17-1. *Pre-op routine—a flowchart.*

On the morning of surgery, you are expected to be at the hospital two to three hours early. Bring any post-op braces, Darco shoe, crutches, or other devices that you were given by your doctor to bring to the hospital. After completing the paperwork, you will be taken to the anesthesia waiting area. In most settings, it is located close to the operating room.

In the waiting room, an IV will be started to give you fluids through the veins. It is a point of entry for sedation, relaxation, and/or anesthesia. The operating room nurse should know about any allergies, dentures, contact lenses, artificial prostheses (including total joint replacements) or other metal you may have in your body. Then you wait for surgery.

ANESTHESIA

Anesthesia is a special medicine to numb the area of surgery. It is a critical aspect of surgery. The choice of anesthetic is determined by your medical health, the surgeon, and the type of surgery planned. You actually participate in the decision after being apprised of the risks and expectations by your doctor and the anesthesiologist in the initial interview.

Anesthesia for Foot Surgeries

There are five types of anesthesia for foot surgeries:

1. **Local injection or toe block.** The nerves around the surgery area are anesthetized by an injection of Xylocaine (type of novocaine).

2. **Regional block.** The nerves around the ankle are injected in such a way as to numb the whole foot.

3. **Epidural block.** The back around the nerves (not in spinal cord) is injected with Xylocaine, novocaine, or similar nerve-numbing medicine. It is the type of anesthetic often used with pregnancy/delivery.

4. **Spinal block.** An injection of anesthetic agent (form of novocaine) into the spinal canal, but not into the spinal cord.

5. **General anesthesia.** The entire body is anesthetized by injecting various medicines (through your IV) to put you to sleep during surgery.

The risk of death from any form of anesthesia is 1 in 10,000 or .0001 percent. Each form has advantages and disadvantages as shall be explained below. This should dispel some "old wives' tales" you may have heard about anesthetics.

Local or Toe Anesthesia

This form of anesthesia offers several advantages:

1. It is the most simple and risk-free anesthesia that can be administered. If toe surgery is planned that does not extend to the base of the toe, an injection just around the toe provides excellent numbness.

2. Fewer needle sticks which means less discomfort for the patient.

3. Used for removing pins or non-deepseated screws from patients.

Among the disadvantages of local or toe anesthesia is the type of allergic reaction which can happen after any type of anesthesia. That is why you must tell your doctor of any unusual reactions including excessive nausea, vomiting, hives or rashes, or pulmonary problems related to previous anesthesia. The "guilty" medicine needs to be identified to ensure that it won't be used again.

Some people are allergic to Xylocaine or derivatives generally used in ankle or local blocks. Most anesthesiologists use such medicine in a preservative-free form to minimize reactions. A previous reaction may have been to the Xylocaine used by a dentist or other medical professional that had preservatives in it. This type of medicine is more cost-effective and common than the form without preservatives.

Medical professionals are well trained in handling allergic reactions to minimize any risk to the patient. If a true reaction to the pure Xylocaine (or derivatives) is known in advance, the anesthesiologist or a dermatologist will do a skin patch test using other forms of this medicine. The goal is to find one that does not cause a reaction. As long as the test is done with trained professionals and there is emergency equipment available, this test procedure is acceptable.

Ankle Block Anesthesia

This is an excellent anesthesia for any toe or midfoot surgery, including some less complex hindfoot surgery. It is by far the first choice of anesthesia for most patients.

Ankle block anesthesia has several advantages:

1. No urinary retention complications.

2. Since it involves injecting a different type of medicine (Marcaine versus Xylocaine or novocaine) into the affected area, the duration of the pain relief is prolonged. This means a much more comfortable first night after surgery. Sometimes the surgeon will perform an ankle block just before the case is completed, even when other anesthesia has been used. This is done to secure longer pain relief after the patient wakes up.

3. No significant bowel, bladder, heart, or lung side effects are associated with this anesthesia.

The main disadvantage of this type of anesthesia is having to use several needle injections to numb the appropriate nerves. To compensate for this discomfort, an anesthesiologist may give you an I.V. sedation to relax you during the minute or two it takes to give the injections.

There are no significant complications from ankle block, unless an inadvertent injection of the nerve itself occurs. Good techniques should eliminate such risk. Even then, lasting effect from injecting a nerve is rare.

Unfortunately, ankle block cannot be used in ankle or more major hindfoot surgeries, because adequate numbing cannot be assured.

Many surgeons use a tourniquet around the patient's ankle for ankle block anesthesia to help eliminate bleeding. Some discomfort from the tourniquet may be experienced, but the sedation medicine should take care of the problem.

Spinal/Epidural Anesthesia

Techniques in spinal anesthesia have been vastly improved. Here are some unique advantages:

1. Quick onset of action. It effectively paralyzes the muscles and is predictable as well.

2. Lesser chance of leg blood clots (deep venous thrombosis).

3. Less postoperative nausea and vomiting.

4. Very small needle is used to inject the medicine.

5. The medicine has no preservatives which eliminates many adverse reactions.

6. Reduced rate of spinal headaches which used to be a major complaint from patients about this form of anesthesia. Headache in the over sixty-age population is rare (less than .5 percent)—two percent for patients under age sixty. The age/complication difference is likely due to the relative increase in tissue stiffness in older patients. This limits the spread of the anesthetic. The central nervous system of older patients is also less reactive to these medicines than younger patients.

7. Less post-op bowel (intestinal) paralysis called ileus. This condition generally results in a distended (swollen) abdomen or belly, making it easy to diagnose.

The main disadvantage of spinal anesthesia is the potential risk of urinary retention because the nerves controlling the muscles of the bladder and the bladder tube sphincter are numbed. Most narcotics for pain like morphine or Demerol also contribute to urinary tract blockage.

During surgery you are given a specified amount of fluid through the vein. This fluid accumulates in the bladder which fails to communicate the sensation of being full due to the numbed nerves. The bladder nerves and muscles can become stretched out, causing a temporary malfunction. For this reason, in long surgical cases that use a lot of fluid or blood transfusions, a foley (tube) catheter is placed in the bladder. This facilitates decompression of the bladder before the stomach becomes stretched.

While you are in the hospital, the medical staff checks you for stomach distention and limits your fluids. If you appear overly distended, they catheterize you before you are discharged to give your nervous system extra time to "wake up." You should limit the amount of your fluid intake before surgery so that you do not contribute to this post-op condition. Once you have voided your bladder adequately, do not feel distended, and start to feel hungry, your nerves have most likely returned to normal. Then you can eat and drink as usual.

After being discharged from outpatient surgery, you may still have a urinary retention problem. If you begin to experience increasing stomach distention and/or abdominal pain and can't urinate (or can only produce a small amount), you need to return to the emergency room immediately. Don't wait for overdistention to occur. In males, prostate enlargement (BPH) is not uncommon. Men with this condition are at a significantly higher risk for this post-op urinary retention problem than women.

Epidural anesthesia does not work in about five percent of patients. This requires additional anesthesia either in the form of a local injection or general anesthesia.

General Anesthesia

In most long and complicated surgeries, this form of anesthesia may be the proper choice. If you have significant anxieties or fears about the surgery which the doctor cannot relieve, then going to sleep may be the best option. That way, you won't have any memory of the procedure.

General anesthesia is also indicated over epidural or spinal anesthesia if you have any bleeding tendency, pernicious anemia, infection-causing fever, generalized sickness, or a neurological disorder like multiple sclerosis. In the latter cases, local anesthesia may confuse your already confused nerves even more. In addition, if you have severe back arthritis or have had back surgery in the area where the epidural or spinal needle is to be inserted, general anesthesia is a better choice. Most surgeries on the abdomen above the belly button, the chest, shoulder, back, and neck cannot be adequately numbed with spinal or epidural blocks. These usually require general anesthesia.

There are obvious disadvantages to general anesthesia. The medications tend to cause more nausea or occasional post-operative vomiting.

Insertion of the breathing (endotracheal) tube required for this anesthesia may cause some broncho (lung tube) spasm, which can increase the risk of postoperative pneumonia and set off an asthmatic attack if you already have asthma.

POSTOPERATIVE PROCEDURES

What should you be doing after surgery? Like the pre-op routines, after surgery you need to follow several crucial steps for speedy (and lasting) recovery. First, most forefoot surgeries (bunions, hammertoes) and less serious ankle or hindfoot surgeries are done as outpatient procedures. This means you are cleared to go home once your doctor and the anesthesiologist or supervisory medical personnel determine that you are medically stable to do so. You are very likely given crutches, a walker, or a wheelchair, depending on your limitations. You'll find preoperative training with these devices quite helpful.

Once at home, it is critical to keep foot and leg elevated above your heart at all times, except when using the bathroom. This is especially true for the acute swelling period of the first seven to ten days after surgery. Ice should be applied to the surgical area fifteen minutes at a time every hour for the first six hours. Then use it four to six times a day for the next several days. DON'T USE HEAT under any circumstances!

Common Pain Medications

In terms of pain medications used postoperatively, Tylenol #3, Percoset, Darvocet N 100, and Motrin are the most common. Sometimes an antibiotic is given for one to two days after surgery to help prevent infection. A compression dressing is also applied to the wound and can become too tight. You can carefully loosen the Ace wrap without removing the bandages. Some blood seepage is normal. Significant pain or numbness can also develop after the anesthetic has worn off. This is a red flag which means you need to call your doctor.

Remember, the time to learn about your surgery, the procedures used, expectations, and possible complications is BEFORE, not after, you have it! As we stressed earlier, you should have a clear understanding of your case and a good comfort level with your doctor before the operation.

IN A NUTSHELL

In this chapter, we have alerted you to standard surgical preparations in elective foot surgery and the role of anesthesia in this important procedure. As a patient, you have the right to know the plan, the expectations, and answers to whatever question is of interest or concern to you before surgery. So in a way you are a participant in the planning of the surgical process.

Remember the important steps to take the day before surgery, the evening before surgery, and the morning of surgery as part of the pre-op routine. You should follow your doctor's orders in this important preparation process. Post-op procedures are also critical for your speedy and lasting recovery.

TERMS TO REMEMBER

Anesthesia: A special medicine to numb the area of surgery.

Ankle block anesthesia: See toe block anesthesia.

Epidural anesthesia: The back around the nerves (not in spinal cord) is injected with a nerve-numbing medicine.

Foley catheter: A tube placed in the bladder to allow urination.

Ileus: Post-op bowel paralysis.

Regional anesthesia: Nerves around the ankle are injected in such a way as to numb the whole foot.

Sphincter: Muscular opening to the bladder tube.

Spinal anesthesia: An injection of anesthetic agent into the spinal canal, but not into the spinal cord.

Toe block anesthesia: Local anesthesia/injection; the nerves around the surgery area are anesthetized by an injection.

PART V

Old Age
Foot Problems

CHAPTER 18

Geriatric Foot Problems

INTRODUCTION

There is no question, it's tough growing old. Certainly it's not for the "faint of heart"! If you hear people complain, "my feet hurt", "my eye glasses seem to weigh two pounds", "I get more exercise getting up at night than I do all day long", "my fat is mostly in my belly, not where I need it", and so on, you know they are definitely in a mature phase of life. This falls under an area called geriatrics.

Geriatrics is a branch of medicine that treats problems related to old age and aging, including senility. Geriatric medicine is a special field, requiring a team effort similar to the care of diabetic patients. When old age actually begins and how one determines it is pretty subjective. One has to consider both chronological and physiological age. A person can have an aged skeletal system (bones that can get arthritis), but a circulation system (heart and the rest) comparable to someone much younger.

No one can help growing old. The trick to this inevitable phase in life is to stay physically healthy and mentally alert. Talk out your problems and stay in touch with your doctor.

Lifestyle, attitude, mental stimulation, and physical activity are additional factors that determine how old is "old".

According to the U.S Census Bureau, there were thirty million American adults over the age of sixty-five in 1988—a number expected to increase to forty million by the year 2000. Studies also have shown that 80 percent of people over age fifty will have foot problems. With the increased activity levels being encouraged by the media, the medical community, and society in general, the severity of these problems is expected to get worse. Yet in the institutionalized older population, a fifty percent reduction in foot problems has been attributed primarily to reduced activity.

KEY PROBLEMS TO ADDRESS

Regardless of the reason, our older population has special psychological and physiological problems that physicians and health professionals need to address. Among the *psychological* problems are:

- **Fear of loss of independence.** Sudden retirement or the reality of growing old affects people in different ways. For example, many senior citizens begin to walk daily for fear of losing use of their feet. Walking, dancing, and socializing are also good therapy, as they promote belonging and feeling good and useful.

- **Financial fears.** It is estimated that 12 percent of the elderly are below the poverty level. With shrinking social security benefits, the average senior citizen has to rely on other sources for support. This is especially critical for senior citizens with physical problems or serious illness.

- **Fear of getting sick.** There is no question that the older a person gets, the more likely the body (and the mind) becomes vulnerable to a variety of physical problems. An active person with a full-time commitment to work and family has quite an adjustment to make after suddenly retiring. Those who do not maintain a level of activity to bridge the transition find themselves with plenty of time to dwell on their body, the likelihood of diseases such as cancer, and what the future might hold for them. This in itself can bring depression, the feeling of no longer being wanted, and the like.

Among the *physical* concerns are:

- **Increased arthritis.** Arthritis surfaces more readily among the elderly, especially those with a genetic history of the disease. This is a valid reason for concern, as it can be disabling if left untreated.

- **Loss of flexibility, coordination, and endurance.** The fact that such problems can occur is the reason for working with the elderly to maintain regular physical exams and monitor their state of health more closely

- **Loss of bone strength (osteoporosis).** As people grow older, the bone structure loses strength and pliability. Bone fractures occur much more readily and are more complex. As a result, one's lifestyle, type of exercise, and mental state has to change.

- **Increased vascular disease.** This shows its ugly teeth more clearly among the elderly and can be more than a nuisance. Activity level is limited because of poor blood supply to the legs. As a result, additional secondary problems develop, including weak or osteoporotic bones, loss of endurance, cardiac fitness, and mental stress.

- **Increased peripheral neuropathies.** Neuropathic arthropathy is a common foot and ankle problem that can have serious consequences, especially with the diabetic elderly.

- **Other increased diseases.** These include possible heart problems, lung problems such as shortness of breath, eyesight problems, diabetes, and cancer—all of which tend to show up more readily among the elderly.

With all these concerns, you can understand how important it is for you and your doctor to communicate clearly the nature of your concern, the importance of following doctor's orders, and undergoing the kinds of tests and procedures that will ensure a healthy and happy lifestyle. You should also tell your doctor about the importance of exercise for your general well-being. Any exercise should be tailored for you to include the constraints imposed by the aging process.

CONDITIONS ENCOUNTERED

In this chapter, the focus is on special foot and leg problems that are more prevalent in the aging population. There are several common conditions that the elderly encounter; each condition deserves special attention:

- **Skin problems** have many faces. A common condition is dry skin with fissuring, secondary eczema, or infection. Nail fungus infections do occur, but thickened, hard-to-care-for brittle nails (onychogryphosis) are more common. Experience also indicates that poor eyesight, loss of joint and leg mobility, and loss of manual dexterity often lead to poor or neglected nail care. When that occurs, it leads to more infections, in-grown toenails, or dermatitis. The bottom line is that skin strength deteriorates in the older population which makes this group more susceptible to injury and skin problems.

- **Normal aging,** which causes the loss of connective tissue elasticity and reduced cellular function. Eventually, this leads to the loss of heel and forefoot shock absorbing pads. Metatarsalgia and heel pain are quite common as we age, mainly because of the loss of fatty cell cushioning. See figure 18-1.

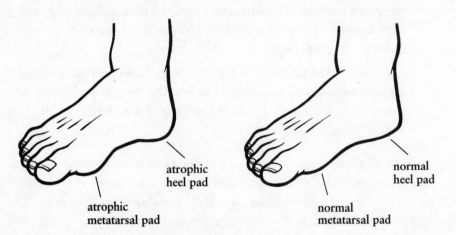

atrophic
heel pad

atrophic
metatarsal pad

normal
heel pad

normal
metatarsal pad

FIGURE 18-1. *Metatarsal pad and heel pad*

- **Changes in foot structure.** It is natural for our foot structure to change as we grow old. Our forefoot widens, flattens, and may even lengthen. As a result, shoe-fitting problems become more significant. Poor fit causes or promotes symptoms in already existing bunions, hammertoes, soft corns, bunionettes, and so on. The supporting arch tendons (posterior tibial tendons) also have a tendency to fail or rupture, leading to further arch pain symptoms, a worsening of bunions, and/or the secondary symptoms mentioned in earlier chapters.

- **Loss of bone mass (osteoporosis)** begins rather quickly in women at the cessation of menstruation and five years thereafter, before it slows down. In contrast, men lose bone mass, but at a slower rate. By age seventy-five, men catch up with women. When you combine weakened bones with normal loss of physical strength, endurance, coordination, and eyesight problems, the result is more injuries, particularly fractures.

- **Increased incidence of leg/foot stiffness and arthritis.** With loss of flexibility comes the risk of falling, loss of ability to do quality activities, and an increased chance of fractures.

- **Vascular problems,** either from arterial blockage or from chronic venous disease. Such problems may lead to ulcers, ischemia (death of tissue), or secondary severe infections.

- **Leg swelling** from vein or lymph disease which often leads to stiffness and symptoms similar to arthritis.

- **Decreased circulation and weaker soft bones.** When this happens, you can expect wounds to heal more slowly and become more easily infected than ever before.

In addition, one needs to consider the interplay among these problems and others that complicate the treatment process.

Self-Help Treatment

One of the most important sources of self-help is the immediate family. Other sources such as support groups and close friends help the older population keep their minds and bodies more fit. They also assist in the early detection of disease. In prescribing suggestions and procedures to consider, the following are ideas worth following:

- **Put medicine away in a separate compartment.** Keep a list of your current medications readily available for reference and cross-reference. Many senior citizens afflicted with multiple physical problems seem to have a mini-pharmacy of their own, with no organization or order to the variety of drugs they use. Worse yet are medicines that have long expired or are no longer necessary. They should be disposed of or placed in a separate cabinet. In any case, family members need to know where medicines are kept, who the doctors are, and how to reach certain doctors for immediate help.

- **Notify your doctors what medicines you're taking.** Doctors don't like surprises, especially when dealing with serious diseases that require close monitoring. If you switch doctors, notify the new doctor what medicine you have been taking and for how long.

- **Don't perform your own surgery on areas that pose the risk of infection.** For example, we cautioned in chapter 10 about the dangers of trimming calluses or corns if you are a diabetic. Any infection is potentially serious and needs to be evaluated rightaway.

  Related to this point is the importance of having your nails cared for by a family member or a knowledgeable professional every few months. Proper nail care and methods are described in the nail section of this book.

- **Wear proper shoes and maintain frequent check of foot size.** It is important to watch for redness or signs of irritation on your feet. Jogging shoes are excellent shock-absorbing shoes for walking and everyday use. They also provide more stability or security for an unsteady gait.

- **Consider foot cushioning** that will give your feet the best possible comfort. For example, Spenko or sorbathane shoe inserts can make all the difference in foot cushioning.

Vera, a seventy-two-year-old woman in good health except for a minor heart problem, came to my office with severe foot pain and swelling. She had just returned from a sight-seeing trip to New England and had gone to an emergency room there for her problem. They found no fracture and told her to see an orthopedist.

Vera had osteoporosis and a stress fracture in her foot. She was given Darco shoe and crutches and was to see her medical doctor for estrogen therapy, calcium and vitamin D supplements. After menstruation stops, there is estrogen loss which weakens bones. Estrogen therapy is best started as soon as menstruation ends but can benefit the older population as well. Adequate calcium and vitamin D are also important for bone strengthening.

As Vera recovered, she was started on a gradual working program, wearing good walking shoes and using one- or two-pound wrist weights to strengthen her arms. She joined a mall walking group and continued to enjoy the walking and companionship. A mall provides an even surface and safe environment. She has had no new problems with stress fractures.

- **Be careful to wear the right kinds of socks or stockings.** Cotton or wool stockings are better at absorbing moisture than synthetic ones like nylon socks. Stockings should *not* constrict at the top. If leg swelling or significant varicose veins are present, you'd be better off wearing short leg Jobst (compression) stockings. These are especially helpful when you are on your feet for any length of time. They also dramatically reduce the aching in your legs or feet.

- **Get into the habit of an exercise program** tailored to your state of health and one that can be monitored by your doctor. A healthy attitude toward regular exercise means a healthy body and a functioning mind. You feel younger and can add satisfaction and happiness to your life.

Exercise Programs

For the elderly, choosing the right exercise program is critical. The best advice is to work with your doctor on a program that you enjoy and that benefits your body. Some exercise programs include swimming, running, and use of health clubs where a variety of exercise equipment is available.

Swimming is an aerobic exercise that offers all the land aerobics without stress to your joints. Water helps decrease stress on bones, but offers eighteen times the resistance of air. Many local community centers have supervised water, walking, or aerobic programs. These are appropriate and inexpensive ways to start exercising.

Health clubs offer a variety of exercise programs and equipment to support them. Most of the better clubs have equipment uniquely suited to the elderly. Before exercising, you need to be evaluated and have instructions from the health club trainer or specialist about the equipment, process, and duration of the exercise. Check out the club and make sure there is enough supervision and attention given to your needs.

Walking program. Walking is an excellent exercise for the elderly and an appropriate alternative to running, as less stress is put on the joints. Using a track in preference to the road is a good idea and safer. Adding one- or two-pound weights to your wrists can improve the cardiovascular workout.

Running/jogging program. Running or jogging is not an activity for everyone. There is always the glamour of seeing runners or joggers go by at an impressive pace or speed. If you enjoy this type of exercise, be careful to check your state of health and have your doctor approve a supervised program that will allow you to break into such high energy exercise without unnecessary risks. In any case, try to jog on dirt rather than pavement or other hard surfaces. It is easier on your bones and ankles.

What About Diet?

It is a fact that the intestinal tract of the elderly does not absorb as well as it once did. If obesity or being overweight is a problem, supervised dieting can make a difference. Calcium (1-1.5 grams) and vitamin D supplement (400,000 units) is a recommended daily dose to supplement your diet and help counteract osteoporosis. Be sure to check with your doctor, however, for any contra-indications.

When it comes to dieting, the worst thing is to resort to over-the-counter diet fads. Most of these diet programs have side effects that you should be warned about. They could affect your blood pressure, upset your stomach, promote dizziness, upset your bowel movement, and the like. The best way to diet is to have a balanced meal and exercise regularly.

Dealing with Calluses and Pressure Areas on Your Foot

For the elderly, we caution against use of any chemicals to remove calluses or bunions, as they cause burns, blisters, or skin ulcers. Care must be taken to use warm soaks, making sure that the water is not hot enough to cause burns. Moleskin, hammertoe pads, or tube foam is available over-the-counter to help relieve pressure areas on your foot.

Related to this aspect of self-help is the importance of walking on dry floors, well-lighted stairs, and an otherwise safe environment. Avoid unnecessary use of stairs or walking barefoot.

Medical Treatment

Depression is a common problem among the elderly. In some cases, they require psychological as well as medical treatment. The important point is to look into the core of the problems besetting you and then approach it in an objective, realistic way. For example, more and more overweight people, having tried in vain to control their weight, often end up in frustration and eventual depression. This, in turn, promotes weight gain and the resulting "yo-yo" effect of dieting.

There are excellent support groups and antidepressant medications. It would help to share certain problems with family members, who could form a reliable support group. Loss of sleep or appetite and frequent mood changes may be indicators of depression. Heed such signs and look at ways to prevent depression from happening.

Older people are generally reluctant to ask questions or talk about deep-seated depressions. Hidden fears or concerns that have gone unchecked for years take time to alleviate. Remember that in any treatment, open communication or discussion is the most critical requirement for treating such problems. An effective support group promotes communication, identification, and self-esteem. Serious problems of depression are best handled by a psychologist, psychiatrist, or a geriatric doctor.

In terms of medical treatment of the older foot, here are some ideas:

- Basic arthritis treatment should be used. The simple NSAIDs are often effective but need to be monitored because side effects and drug interactions are more common in the elderly.

- If there is recurrent skin breakdown or ulcers, simple toe surgery with low risk anesthesia should be considered before the problem becomes more serious.

- Consider the occasional help of a physical therapist. A short course of a variety of more sophisticated modalities like ultrasound, ionotophoresis, a TENS unit, and gentle specific exercises may do wonders. This is also useful for treating depression as well as physical symptoms and imbalances.

- For the medically impaired such as stroke patients or diabetics, the tendency for contracture and inability to place the foot correctly on a surface is much higher. Physical therapy, appropriate pressure-relieving shoes, braces, or other devices are frequently critical.

Surgical Treatment

Most foot problems of the elderly have been present for a long time and most of these patients have no interest in major surgical procedures. Other treatments should be tried first. The trend toward living a longer productive life, safer anesthesia, and more sophisticated and simpler surgical techniques, however, make elective surgery more viable and safer than ever before. Most of today's elective surgeries are relatively low risk and successful. For example, vascular surgery to save a limb now has a high success rate in all ages.

Anyone electing to have surgery should consider the immobilization and adjustments that follow surgery. Older patients with arthritis tend to become stiff, especially when placed in casts. In addition, with mobilization, osteoporosis is made worse and can cause additional problems. As a result, a simpler procedure is usually tried to correct foot problems, since the older patient puts less demand on the feet.

In any event, when it comes to surgery, all the medical risks need to be considered. If surgery is required, anesthesia selection is very important, because complications increase and medications interact and need to be carefully monitored. See chapter 17 on foot surgery and anesthesia.

Many fractures of the ankle or foot in the active older population warrant surgery. This is especially true if the joint is broken or out of place. The methods used to fix the fracture are more extensive in order to avoid the use of casts or braces. The opposite is true in the inactive elderly. Fractures are often left alone even though there is an increased chance of arthritis or limited movement. The activity level, mental status, and bone strength of the patient are factors in making this decision.

IN A NUTSHELL

Old age is inevitable, bringing with it its own share of foot and other problems. Geriatrics treats medical problems related to old age. Your job as a patient is to work on the causes of the problems that make you physically ill or mentally depressed. You should learn to communicate your concerns to your doctor and close family, friends, or a support group. Don't dwell on the weak parts of your body. If you stay in shape through exercise and regular checkups and active by doing the things that bring you satisfaction and pleasure, old age begins to lose its potency. Instead, you can add years to your life and life to your years.

DOCTOR'S CORNER:
QUESTIONS AND ANSWERS

What can I do to help prevent my elderly mother from developing foot problems?

You or her caregiver should assist your mother in a daily check of her feet for redness, swelling, blisters, and so on. It is very important to ensure that she is wearing proper, well-fitting shoes. Remind her to elevate her legs and avoid crossing them to prevent swelling. Provide her with a moisturizer for her skin and make sure she has proper nail care. She needs to avoid self "surgery" by trimming corns and calluses. This should be done by a health care professional.

As I get older, I find that I can't wear most of my shoes because they are too tight. Why is this happening?

As you age, the ligament in your arch and toes loosens and your feet become wider and even longer. For this reason, it is important to have your feet measured for size every time you buy shoes. Your shouldn't wear any shoes that feel too tight because any foot problems like bunions, etc., will worsen from ill-fitting shoes. Aging also reduces the natural cushioning on your heels and the balls of your feet. Your shoes need more cushioning and the addition of soft orthotics for shock absorption and comfort might help, as well.

I am eighty-three years old. I have a bunion on my big toe which doesn't bother me, but I have a severe hammertoe on my second toe. I can't wear any shoes comfortably—even lace up walking shoes. My doctor recommended amputation of my second toe, which seems extreme. What should I do?

Your condition is not uncommon in the older population. You have adapted to your bunion and it is not painful but your second toe is very disabling. Correcting the bunion and the hammertoe is a much bigger operation than amputating the second toe. Correcting the hammertoe alone will not be permanent, since your bunion will make it recur.

Because of your age and other medical factors, amputation of the second toe is a good procedure and won't limit your walking ability. This is a doctor/patient decision, and you need to feel comfortable with it before you proceed.

TERMS TO REMEMBER

Geriatrics: A branch of medicine that treats problems related to old age and aging, including senility.

Onchyogryphosis: Brittle nails.

Osteoporosis: Loss of bone strength.

Glossary of Terms

Accessory navicular: The enlarged anatomical variation of the navicular bone which appears as a bony prominence in the arch. The posterior tibial tendon attaches here.

Achilles tendinitis: Inflammation or microscopic tears of the calf tendon.

Achilles tendon: The heel cord which is an extension of the calf muscle and controls the ability to rise on the toes; a large tendon located in the back of the ankle.

Adduct: To move a body component (e.g the foot) toward the center of the body.

Alphabet exercise: An exercise, where the sufferer "writes out" the alphabet in the air with his/her ankle to stimulate ankle motion in all directions.

Analgesic: A medicine to relieve pain.

Anesthesia: A special medicine to numb the area of surgery.

Anesthesiologist: See glossary of medical specialists.

Ankle block anesthesia: See toe block anesthesia.

Ankle circles: An exercise to maintain ankle and foot motion; turning the foot slowly clockwise, then counterclockwise, and gradually increasing size of circles as pain and swelling permit.

Ankle joint: Top of the talus and the end of the two leg bones of the foot.

Ankle orthroscopy: A surgical procedure, where the scar tissue or small chip is removed from the ankle by an arthroscope through small incisions.

Ankle pump: Moving the ankle back and forth in a pumping motion; an exercise used with acute soft tissue injuries, including sprains.

Ankylosing spondylitis: Mainly hip and back arthritis, but resistent heel pain and MTP joint inflammation may be present.

Anterior tibial muscle: A muscle that allows you to move your foot up toward your shin.

Arch: A curved part of the underside of the foot.

Arch ligament (plantar fascia): A band of strong fibers or the ligament that connects the heel to the toes and runs along the arch of the foot.

Arteriogram: A test where dye is injected into a leg artery to show a picture of the arteries in order to determine the circulation and/or areas of blockage.

Arthritis: A disease that has many forms and involves inflamed joint lining (synovitis) and the disruption of shock absorbing cartilage that covers the ends of bones at the joints.

Arthrodesis (fusion): The elimination of a specific joint or foot motion by locking bones together to gain stabilization and eliminate pain.

Arthroscopy: Small incision surgery using a small tube lens system that is inserted to allow visualization of the entire joint via a small camera. Small surgical instruments inserted into tiny incisions are used to perform the surgery.

Articular cartilage: Shock absorbing elastic tissue covering the ends of bone.

Athlete's foot: A fungus infection of the foot, usually found on the sole between the toes or the sole of the foot.

Atrophy: The loss of normal muscle size, appearance, and function. It occurs rapidly when muscle is not used or is injured.

Avulsion fracture: The pulling off of a piece of bone during injury that is not considered a significant fracture and is usually treated as a sprain.

Blister: A fluid-filled sac that forms as a result of friction.

Bone scan: A special x-ray obtained by injecting dye that highlights injured or diseased bone areas.

Bone spur: A bony outgrowth indicating arthritis or bone irritation.

Bowleg (genu varum): The knees are spread apart while the ankles and feet are close together. It may or may not be associated with additional torsion problems.

Bromohidrosis: A term meaning smelly feet.

Bunion: A bump, abnormality, or deviation of the big toe joint that is misaligned and caused by abnormal pressures.

Bunionette: A bunion of the fifth toe (pinkie).

Bursitis: An inflamed bursa which is the sac filled with synovial fluid over a joint that helps decrease friction.

Calcaneous: The great bone of the heel and the largest bone in the foot.

Calcaneous fracture: Heel fracture.

Callus: A thickening of the skin caused by recurring friction or pressure on the skin caught between bone and an adjacent firm surface like a shoe or the floor.

Cartilage: Fibrous elastic material covering the ends of bones which allows joints to move freely with minimal friction and aids in shock absorption.

Causalgia syndrome: See RSD.

Cavus foot (pes cavus): An abnormally high arch foot which is usually stiff and provides poor shock absorption; a foot with a high arch.

Charcot: Degenerative disorder of the central and peripheral nervous system of the foot; an early breakdown of ligaments and tendons leading to deformities and joint dislocations.

Charcot arthropathy: A progressive bone, ligament, and tendon destructive disease that is related to neuropathy. It can result in severe foot deformity. It most commonly occurs in diabetics, but can occur with other abnormal nerve problems.

Claudication: See intermittent claudication.

Claw toe: A combination of hammertoe and mallet toe, caused by abnormal pressures or buckling at both toe joints.

Closed fracture: A broken bone with no resulting break in the skin.

Club foot (talipes equinovarus): In this birth defect, the heel cord, ankle, arch ligament, and joints are extremely contractive (tight), causing the toes and heels to point down and inwards. The forefoot (metatarsal) bones also point abnormally inward.

Coagulation: The clotting of blood.

Colitis: A bowel inflammation.

Comminuted fracture: A bone broken in several places that usually requires surgery using plates, screws, or pins to repair.

Congenital dislocated hips: A birth defect of abnormal hip joints where the ball is dislocated from the socket. It requires early identification and treatment for best results.

Contact dermititis: Allergic reaction to shoe materials or chemical additives in the rubber.

Contusion: A bruising injury that does not break the skin.

Corn: Like a callus, but usually found between or on top of the toes. They may be hard or soft thickened skin.

Cryopump: For physical therapy, an intermittently inflating pump that uses cold and compression to reduce swelling.

Cryosurgery: Surgery using freezing techniques like liquid nitrogen.

Cuboid: A pyramid-shaped bone on the edge of the foot between the heel and the bones leading to the fourth and fifth toes.

Curly toe: A toe that curls under an adjacent toe.

Custom-molded orthotics: A foot support of various materials, made from a special mold of the patient's foot, used for cushioning or altering foot motions and stresses.

Debridement: The surgical removal of infected or dead (necrotic) tissue and foreign matter.

Dermatologist: See glossary of medical specialists.

Dermis: The vascular layer of the inner skin which contains sweat glands and fat cells.

Diabetes: A system disease or disorder caused by the body's inability to transport sugar from blood to the cells; related to a deficiency or inefficient use of insulin.

Diabetes mellitus: Medical term for diabetes.

Displaced fracture: A fracture where the broken bones are out of normal position.

Distal joints: Joints in the toe closest to the nail.

Dorsi flexion: Moving the toes up—a motion to the ankle joint.

Dyshidrosis: Excessive smelling tendency.

Edema: Swelling caused from an excess of fluid.

EMG: Electromyographic study to diagnose muscle function abnormality, using electrodes on the skin or fine gauge needles in the muscle.

Endocrinologist: See glossary of medical specialists.

Epidermis: The outer layer of skin which is non-vascular.

Epidural anesthesia: Injection of the back around the nerves (not in spinal cord) with a nerve-numbing medicine.

Erythematosis: Redness, indicating inflammation from infection or injury.

Eversion: Moving the foot away from the midline.

Extensor muscle: A muscle that allows you to straighten your toes.

Extensor tendinitis: Inflammation of the extensor tendon.

Extensor tendons: Tendons on the top of the foot that lift (extend) the toes off the floor.

Extra depth shoes: Shoes that have more space in the forefoot for accommodating deformities of the foot and toes.

Family physician: See glossary of medical specialists.

Femur: The thigh bone with the top end making up part of the hip joint.

Fibula: The smaller of the two bones between the ankle and the knee.

Fissure: A small crack in the skin frequently related to dry skin conditions or neuropathies. Cracks serve as entry points for infection.

Flare: Curve of a shoe.

Flat foot: A foot that lacks or has a decreased arch.

Flexible accommodative orthotics: Orthotics made from a mold of the foot used to relieve the diabetic foot or a tight foot; shock absorbing.

Flexor muscle: A muscle that allows you to bend your toes.

Flexor tendons: Tendons that are attached to muscles that curl the toes toward the floor.

Flexor tenosynovitis: Inflammation of the flexor tendon and its surrounding sheath.

Foley catheter: A tube placed in the bladder to decompress the bladder and allow urination.

Forefoot: Ball and toes of the foot; anterior foot.

Fracture: A break in the normal anatomy of the bone.

Fusion: A surgical procedure where extra bone is used to provide a fixed joint in order to secure a more stable position. See also arthrodesis.

Gait analysis: An approach used for monitoring and observing gait.

Gait cycle: The sequence of movements in walking and running, including heel strike to push off.

Gangrene: Death of tissue from lack of blood supply.

Gerontologist: See glossary of medical specialists.

Gout: A form of arthritis, where excess uric acid forms painful crystals in joints. The big toe is frequently afflicted.

Hallux: The big toe.

Hallux valgus: Bunion of the big toe.

Hallux varus: A condition where the big toe bends in the opposite direction or away from the number two toe.

Hammertoe: A deformed toe that buckles up at the middle toe joint.

Hapad: A cushioned metatarsal pad used to relieve pressure.

Heel and sole lift: A device used in adjusting short leg problems.

Heel bone: The os calcis or calcaneous bone. It is the largest foot bone.

Heel cord (Achilles tendon): The large tendon in the back of the ankle.

Heel counter: The part of the shoe that controls the heel. It is stiff material that supports the heel and outer leather or quarter and prevents the heel from rolling over.

Heel cup (heel cushion): A device to help relieve heel pain by adding shock absorption to the heel and placing it in a better weight bearing position.

Heel flares: A widened heel extending beyond the heel counter. Used with progressing flat foot (pronation) or on the outside of the heel if the ankle is unstable (supination).

Heel pad: The soft tissue of the heel primarily made up of fatty tissue and the primary heel shock absorber.

Heel pain syndrome: Localized or central heel pad tenderness which is the most frequent cause of heel pain.

Heel/sole wedge: Used to change the angle of pressures on the foot, ankle, or knee. It is an angled wedge added to the shoe or placed inside the shoe.

Heel spur: A small bony protrusion from the front of the heel a few millimeters in size where the arch ligament of the foot attaches (plantar fascia).

Heel stabilizer: Extensions of the heel counter on shoes on the medial (inside) or lateral (outside) to keep the heel in a better weight bearing position and help control excess pronation or supination, respectively.

Hematoma: A swelling that contains blood, usually caused by injury.

High arch (pes cavus): See cavus foot.

Hindfoot: Part of the foot that links the ankle joint to the midfoot.

Hoffman procedure: A surgical procedure that requires the removal of the ends of metatarsals.

Hyperglycemia: A condition with an excess of sugar in the blood.

Hypoglycemia: A condition with too little sugar in the blood.

Ileus: Post-op bowel paralysis.

Impingement syndrome: The compression, pinching, and/or irritation of soft tissue—like tendons and ligaments that are under a bony prominence or protrusion.

Index of suspicion: An extra awareness, sensitivity, and knowledge of diseases that are elusive, hard to diagnose, and often overlooked.

Indium study: A special bone scan using indium dye material to identify bone infection (osteomyelitis). The dye is injected into the blood and allowed to circulate; then a picture is obtained.

Infectious disease doctor: See glossary of medical specialists.

Ingrown toenail: The edge of the toenail penetrates the groove of the nail and presses into tissue. It is painful and becomes infected easily.

Insulin: A pancreatic hormone that is necessary for metabolizing carbohydrates and used to control sugar. A lack of this hormone is a major cause of diabetes.

Interdigital neuroma: See Morton's neuroma.

Intermittent claudication: A condition caused by circulation problems that creates pain and cramps in the legs during exercise that is relieved during rest.

Internal femoral torsion: In-turning of the entire leg, including the hips and thighs. The knee caps point inward.

Internal medicine doctor (internist): See glossary of medical specialists.

Interphalangeal joint: The joint between the phalanges or the toe bones.

Inversion: Bringing the big toe toward the midline.

Inversion sprain: The most common ankle sprain caused by twisting inward and injuring the ligaments on the outside of the ankle.

Iontophoresis: A physical therapy technique using electrical currents to carry medicine through intact skin to heal inflammation and control swelling.

Ischemia: Vascular deficiency (lack of circulation) from a blockage of arterial blood flow that results in poor oxygen supply and death of tissue unless circulation is restored.

Joint capsule: The supportive tissue holding the two joint bones together.

Keller procedure: A specific bunion or great toe arthritis operation that removes half of the joint to relieve pressure and/or realign the joint. It is not as commonly used as in the past.

Knock knee (genu valgum): The knees are touching or close together and the feet are spread apart. It may or may not be associated with additional torsion problems.

Lace stay: The reinforced part of the upper shoe that contains the eyelets for laces.

Last: The form over which a shoe is constructed. The most common types are outflare, inflare, or combination lasts.

Lateral: The outside of the foot or leg; the "little toe" side.

Lateral stablizer: Extension of the heel counter on the outside (lateral) may be used in supination problems.

Lesion: An abnormal change in an organ due to injury or disease.

Ligament: Additional supportive structures just outside the joint that provide stability and connect the two joint bones together.

Lipoma: A benign overgrowth of fatty tissue.

Lisfranc joints: Joints located across the foot between the metatarsal bones and the midtarsal bones.

Maceration: A breaking down of skin tissue—often associated with oozing.

Magnetic resonance imaging (MRI): A diagnostic procedure using a complex magnet, radio waves, and atomic nuclei. It is an excellent study to show soft tissue problems (ligaments, tendons, blood vessels).

Mallet toe: A deformed toe that is bent under at the end toe joint.

Medial: The midline or inside of the foot or leg; the "big toe" side of the foot.

Medial stabilizer: Extension of the heel counter to include inside (pronation) problems.

Metatarsal: One of five long bones of the forefoot.

Metatarsal bar: Similar to a rocker sole. It is used for metatarsalgia. The pressure is transferred toward the heel and away from the ball of the foot.

Metatarsalgia: A painful condition, usually on the ball of the foot.

Metatarsal pad: A soft elevated device placed in shoes behind the ball of the foot to relieve pressure from the ball of the foot and relieve metatarsalgia and calluses.

Metatarsal phalangeal (MTP) joint: The joint at the base of the toe close to the web space. It is associated with the ball of the foot.

Metatarsus adductus: A foot deformity that involves the forefoot, not the heel; front part of the foot turning inward at birth. It needs early correction with exercise and sometimes casting or surgery.

Midfoot: Five short bones and the main arch that acts to stabilize and support body weight.

Modified McBride procedure: A soft tissue surgical ligament release and tightening procedure to correct a bunion.

Moleskin: A soft felt used as a skin protector for blisters, calluses, corns, and so on. Sold over-the-counter.

Morton's neuroma: Interdigital neuroma; the most common nerve problem in the foot, usually occurring between the third or fourth toe—occasionally between the second and third toe.

Motor neuropathy: When the nerve supply to muscle is diseased, the muscle does not function and becomes atrophied. Some muscles function better than their opposite partners, causing muscle imbalance. This can cause deformity in the foot. See chapter 7 for nerve problems and the autonomic nervous system.

MRI: See magnetic resonance imaging

MTP: See metatarsal phalangeal joint.

Navicular: A boat-shaped bone in the midfoot.

Nerve conduction velocity: An electrical study which measures the speed of nerve conduction to help diagnose nerve abnormalities. Neither painful nor risky.

Neurologist: See glossary of medical specialists.

Neuroma: A swelling of a nerve associated with inflammation of the nerve or the tissue surrounding the nerve.

Neuropathy: When the nerve supply is diseased, the diseased nerve may cause sensation (feeling) abnormalities, loss of muscle function, or nerve malfunction (poor, sweaty), or all of these.

Night cast: A removable cast that is worn at night to help stretch the heel cord and eliminate heel pain.

NSAID: Nonsteroidal anti-inflammatory medicine: a general term for medicines that treat inflammation, pain, and swelling. Most are prescription medicines, but some are over-the-counter. All can cause side effects, primarily involving the stomach or intestine.

Nutritionist: See glossary of medical specialists.

Occupational therapist: See glossary of medical specialists.

Open fracture: A broken bone that protrudes through the skin.

Opthalmologist: See glossary of medical specialists.

Orthopedic shoe: An off-the-shelf shoe that has more depth and width than a regular shoe.

Orthopedic surgeon: See glossary of medical specialists.

Orthotics: Molded or standard inserts which are placed inside the shoe.

Orthroscopy: A surgical procedure, where scar tissue or small chip is removed from the ankle through small incisions.

Os calcis: The heel bone.

Osteoarthritis: Degenerative or mechanical arthritis; degeneration of the cartilage and bones of joints.

Osteomyelitis: Bone infection. A serious problem and hard to eradicate.

Osteotomies: Realignment of the foot; realignment bone correction. The surgical cutting of bone for realignment and the relief of abnormal pressures causing deformities.

Overpronation: Overflattening of the arch during weight bearing; synonymous with excessive pronation.

Oversupination: An abnormal lateral rotation of the foot during weight bearing.

Pedorthist: See glossary of medical specialists.

Periosteum: The protective membrane made of connective tissue that surrounds bone.

Peripheral neuropathy: A malfunction of the nerve after it has left the spinal cord that causes abnormal sensation and response to pain, sweating, skin temperature; alters muscle functions. It is usually found in diabetics.

Peroneal muscles: Muscles that control the outside of the ankle to prevent ankle sprain and on the outside of the leg to turn the foot outward.

Phalanges (phalanx): A general term for small bones in the toes and fingers.

Phalanx: Singular of phalanges; one of the small bones of the toes.

Physiatrist: See glossary of medical specialists.

Physical therapist: See glossary of medical specialists.

Pigeon-toed turning feet: It may be related to internal femoral torsion, internal tibial torsion, or both.

Pinkie: The fifth toe.

PIP: See proximal interphalangeal joint.

Plantar fascia: The longest ligament in the foot; the main arch ligament that connects the heel to the toes and runs along the arch of the foot.

Plantar fasciitis: An inflamed and strained arch ligament with partial small ruptures that is commonly associated with claw toes and tight heel cords.

Plantar flexion: Moving the toes down to the floor—a motion to the ankle joint.

Plantar pad: The fatty tissue on the ball of the foot which acts as a shock absorber.

Plantar wart: A small infectious wart on the bottom of the foot caused by a virus.

Podiatrist: See glossary of medical specialists.

Popliteal artery: The main artery that supplies the foot with blood.

Posterior tibial muscle/tendon unit: This is the main supporting muscle/tendon unit of the arch. It is located on the inside of the ankle and foot. Shin splints are related to this leg muscle/tendon.

Pronation: The abnormal rolling over to the inside of the foot while weight bearing that in overpronation can flatten the arch and cause the toes to point out instead of straight ahead. Occurs normally during walking, but when done excessively, causes problems.

Prosthesis: An artificial device used to restore lost foot or leg function; that is, an artificial leg or foot.

Prosthetist: See glossary of medical specialists.

Proximal interphalangeal (PIP) joints: The joints in the middle of the toes.

Psoriasis: A condition that shows up as a scaling eruption on several areas of the foot.

Pump bump (retrocalcaneal bursitis): An inflammation of the heel bursa between the Achilles tendon and the heel bone that can be painful when the shoe pushes against it.

Quarter: The back portion of the upper shoe which holds the heel counter and surrounds it.

Regional anesthesia: Nerves around the ankle are injected in a way that numbs the entire foot.

Rehabilitation: A set of exercises or routines designed to return a person to maximum function.

Reiter's syndrome: An infectious disease, showing symptoms such as eye inflammation, genital inflammation/discharge, bowel inflammation, or swollen toe.

Relative rest: Maintaining an activity level that does not add pain to an injured part and allows some motion to it if this motion does not cause pain.

Retrograde massage: Managing an injured area with motion toward the direction of the heart to reduce swelling.

Rheumatoid arthritis: Arthritic disease that starts in the joint lining (synovium) and often progresses to the destruction of cartilage. It is frequently associated with other medical problems.

Rheumatologist: See glossary of medical specialists.

RICE: An acronym for rest, ice, compression, and elevation; a procedure to combat swelling and inflammation.

Rigid orthotics: Special orthotics used in motion control for flexible foot deformity. It is not very shock absorbing.

Rocker sole: A sole that is rocker shaped to allow the foot to roll rather than bend.

RSD: Reflex sympathetic dystrophy; an abnormal nerve response of the autonomic nervous system that is an elusive disease and is often associated with minor injury. Its pain is out of proportion to the injury.

Rupture: The tearing of a tendon or a ligament.

Scoliosis: A noticeable curvature of the spine.

Semi rigid orthotics: Special orthotics that help control abnormal foot motion and provide some shock absorption.

Sensation testing: Recording the patient's responses to show reactions to a range of feeling from light touch to sharp pin prick. The level of sensation is compared to the patient's opposite foot.

Sesamoiditis: Inflammation of the soft tissue surrounding the sesamoid bones of the great toe at the metatarsal pad.

Sesamoids: The two small bones under the great toe metatarsal.

Shank: The part of the shoe that extends from the heel to just before the MTP joints (ball of the foot) and maintains the shoe shape. The shoe breaks or bends just past the shank.

Shin splints: A common generalized painful condition from overstress and overuse that is located along the inside of the leg bone. It needs to be differentiated from stress fracture.

Silastic: Total joint implant of the great toe.

Simple fracture: A cracked or broken nondisplaced bone.

Skew foot: See metatarsal adductus.

Skin ulcers: A break in tissue from pressure that often leads to a breakdown in the underlying tissue. It occurs commonly in diabetics and is hard to heal.

Sole: The bottom of the shoe.

Spenko: Over-the-counter cushion arch support

Sphincter: Muscular opening to the bladder tube.

Spinal anesthesia: An injection of anesthetic agent into the spinal canal, but not into the spinal cord.

Spondylolysis: Arthritis of the back.

Spondylolisthesis: Advanced stage of a back stress fracture.

Sprain: An injury to a ligament involving some degree of tearing that ranges from mild to moderate to severe.

Spur: A bony outgrowth.

Stance: Weight-bearing phase of walking.

Stress fracture: A painful reaction of bone that occurs when the stress applied to it has exceeded the bone's ability to withstand or remodel to that stress.

Subchondral bone: The hard bone just beneath the cartilage that provides support for the cartilage.

Subungual hematoma: Hemorrhage under the nail plate.

Subtaler joint: The joint located between the ankle bone and heel bone.

Sudek's atrophy: See RSD.

Supination: The rolling of the foot to the outside when weight bearing. Oversupination causes a pigeon-toed gait.

Swing phase: The portion of the walking gait cycle while the leg is swinging through the air and is not weight-bearing.

Synovectomy: Surgery to remove an inflamed joint lining that often includes the rerouting of tendons.

Synovial fluid: The lubricating fluid of joints. Excess synovial fluid is produced when inflammation is present.

Synovium: The lining of the joint which produces synovial fluid.

Systemic: Affecting the entire body.

Talus: The anklebone.

Tarsal coalition: A congenital fusion of two of the mid-tarsal bones of the foot. It is often associated with flat feet and becomes symptomatic in adolescence or young adulthood.

Tarsal tunnel: The tunnel formed by ligament tissue through which the major foot nerves run. It is located on the inside (medial) side of the ankle area.

Tendinitis: Inflamed tendon.

Tendon: The tough elastic fibrous tissue that connects muscle to bone.

TENs unit: A low voltage electric stimulus unit which interrupts and treats a pain cycle.

Thermo-molded shoe: Custom shoe made from the mold of the foot.

Tibia: The larger of the two bones between the knee and the ankle.

Tinea pedis: Fungus skin infection.

Tinel: Direct pressure or tapping of a painful nerve area causes tingling and numbness which radiates away from the nerve, usually into the foot and toes but occasionally backward up into the leg.

Toe block anesthesia: Local anesthesia; the nerves around the surgery area are anesthetized by an injection.

Toe box: The front of the shoe (rounded or pointed) that houses toes; the toe portion of the shoe.

Toe spacer: A shoe insert to separate toes—used with bunions, etc.

Toe towel curls: Crunching up a towel or picking up marbles with the toes to help decrease swelling in the forefoot.

Torque: A twisting force.

Torsion: Toe-in or toe-out; hips or legs that turn inward or outward more than normal.

Triple arthrodesis: Surgical fusion of midtarsal and subtaler joints—frequently performed to relieve painful deformed flat foot problems or other hindfoot deformities.

Ulcer: A break in the continuity of tissue; open sore which often leads to a total breakdown of the underlying tissue and becomes infected.

Ultrasound: A physical therapy technique that uses heat from high frequency sound waves to break up scar tissue, increase circulation, and reduce swelling.

Upper shoe: The upper part of the shoe that includes the vamp, laces, toe piece, heel counter, lasts, shank, and liner.

Vamp: The lower part of the upper shoe that is attached to the sole. It takes the most wear.

Vascular surgeon: See glossary of medical specialists.

Wart: A thickened, painful skin caused by a virus that is often mistaken for a callus. A wart has tiny blood supply marks in it.

Wolin's sign: Scar tissue in the ankle.

—— ～ ——

Glossary of Medical Specialists

Anesthesiologist: A physician trained in the administering and handling of all forms of anesthesia and its complications.

Dermatologist: A physician specializing in treating diseases of the skin and its functions.

Endocrinologist: A medical doctor specializing in treating the diseases of the endocrine glands like the thyroid and pituitary glands.

Family physician: A general medical doctor who treats problems and diseases in patients of all ages.

Gerontologist: A medical doctor specializing in treating problems and diseases associated with the older age population.

Infectious disease doctor: A medical doctor who treats infectious diseases caused by bacteria or virus.

Internal medicine doctor (internist): A medical doctor specializing in the diagnosis and treatment of nonsurgical diseases.

Neurologist: Treats all forms of nerve disease and problems of the nervous system. He or she is often trained in EMG and nerve conduction studies.

Nutritionist: A medical professional trained in the study of nutrition and problems related to nutrition.

Occupational therapist: A medical professional who creates activities to promote recovery and rehabilitation after injury or disease.

Opthalmologist: A physician who specializes in the treatment and surgery of diseases and injuries of the eye.

Orthopedic surgeon: A physician who specializes in treatment and surgery of bone and joint injuries, diseases, and problems.

Orthotist: A brace specialist.

Pedorthist: A person trained in the design, manufacture, fit and modification of shoes and related foot appliances as prescribed to alleviate foot pains or disabling conditions.

Physiatrist: A medical doctor who specializes in treating non-operative muscle and skeletal problems who is trained to perform EMG and nerve conduction studies.

Physical therapist: A medical professional trained in the treatment of disease and injury by physical and mechanical means like massage, regulated exercise, water, light, heat, and electricity therapy.

Podiatrist: A doctor of podiatric medicine trained in the care, treatment, and surgery of the foot.

Prosthetist: A professional trained to make and fit braces and artificial limbs.

Rheumatologist: A medical doctor specializing in treating rheumatic disease like rheumatoid arthritis and rheumatic fever.

Vascular surgeon: A physician specializing in the treatment and surgery of disease and injury to the circulatory system.

~

Directory of Associations & Self-Help Organizations

SELF-HELP

Self-Help Center
150 N. Wacker Dr., Suite 900
Chicago, IL 60606
(312) 368-9030

Serves as a clearinghouse for the collection and dissemination of information on all types of self-help groups. Organizes consultancy workshops bringing laymen and professionals together with self-help group representatives. Conducts educational training programs and research on the emergence, functioning, and effectiveness of self-help groups.

Publications: *Directory of Self-Help/Mutual Aid Groups in Illinois*, annually. Also publishes brochures, pamphlets, workbooks, and articles on self-help mutual aid.

DERMATOLOGY

American Academy of Dermatology (AAD)
930 N. Meacham Rd.
Schaumburg, IL 60172-4965
(708) 330-0230

Professional society of medical doctors specializing in skin disease. Conducts educational programs. Provides placement service; compiles statistics.

Publications: *Dermatology World*, monthly. *Dialogues in Dermatology*, audio-tapes. *Journal of the American Academy of Dermatology*, monthly.

American Board of Dermatology (ABD)
Henry Ford Hospital
Detroit, MI 48202
(313) 874-1088

Examining and certifying body. Seeks to assure competent care for patients with cutaneous diseases, via capable representation. Conducts annual comprehensive examination to determine the competent physicians who meet the requirements for examination by the board.

Publications: *Booklet of Information.*

DIABETES

American Diabetes Association (ADA)
National Center
1660 Duke Street
Alexandria, VA 22314
(703)549-1500
(800) ADA-DISC

Physicians and health professional interested in diabetes mellitus. Promotes the free exchange of information about diabetes mellitus by education the public in the early recognition of the disease, the importance of medical supervision in its treatment, and the development of educational methods designed for people with diabetes. Seeks to find a cure for diabetes and improve the lives of all people affected by the condition.

Publications: *Clinical Diabetes*, bimonthly newsletter. Provides scientific information about diabetes and its treatment to the general physician without specialized training in diabetes.

International Diabetic Athletes Association (IDAA)
1931 East Rovey Ave.
Phoenix, AZ 85016
(602)230-8155

Individuals with diabetes and healthcare professionals. Promotes the participation of individuals with diabetes in sports activities. Provides a network and support group for athletes with diabetes. Conducts educational programs to increase self care skills for individuals with diabetes and counseling skills for healthcare professionals. Offers blood sugar screenings; sponsors volunteer services and speakers' bureau.

Publications: *Challenge*, quarterly newsletter.

Juvenile Diabetes Foundation International (JDFI)
432 Park Ave. S.
New York, NY 10016-8013
(212) 889-7575
(800) JDF-CURE

Juvenile diabetics and their families. Provides counseling and support services to juvenile diabetics and their families.

Publications: *Countdown*, quarterly. Also publishes pamphlets and brochures for diabetics, families, medical personnel, and teachers; produces videotapes.

National Diabetes Information Clearinghouse
P.O. Box NDIC
Bethesda, MD 20892
(301)654-3327

Collects and disseminates information on patient education materials and provides technical guidance for the development of materials and programs for diabetes education. Maintains an automated file of brochures, audiovisual materials, books, articles, teaching manuals, fact sheets, and other educational materials. Services are available to health professionals, to people with diabetes and their families, and to the general public.

FOOTWEAR

Footwear Industries of America (FIA)
1420 K St. NW Suite 600
Washington, DC 20005
(202) 789-1420

American manufacturers of footwear and their suppliers, retailers, importers, and distributors. Provides information on all aspects of the industry including marketing, technology, finance, management, statistics, and national affairs.

Publications: Books. *Dictionary of Shoe Industry Terminology. Executive Digest*, monthly. *Footwear Manual*, annually. *U.S. Footwear Industry Directory*, annually.

National Shoe Retailers Association (NSRA)
9861 Broken Land Parkway, Suite 255
Columbia, MD 21046-1151
(410) 381-8282
(800) 673-8446

Trade association representing independent retailers of footwear. Provides services to shoe retailers and offers professional development programs. Seeks to promote wider public understanding of the importance of proper shoe fit to overall health.

Publications: *Shoe Retailing Today*, monthly newsletter; *Business Performance Report*, biannually; *1994–95 Software Directory: Guidelines for Selecting or Upgrading a Computer System for Shoe Retailers.*

Pedorthic Footwear Association
9861 Broken Land Parkway, Ste. 255
Columbia, MD. 21046-1151
(410) 381-1167
(800) 673-8447

National non-profit association representing professionals involved in the design, manufacture, fit and modification of shoes and related foot appliances to alleviate foot pains or disabling conditions. Sponsors educational courses and programs. Seeks to advance public awareness of pedorthics and of the importance of proper footwear fit to physical health.

Publicatons: *Pedoscope*, bimonthly; *Dealing with Diabetes; Ten Points of Proper Shoe Fit; Pedorthics and the Board-Certified Pedorthist; Directory of Pedorthics.*

GERIATRIC

National Association of Professional Geriatric Care Managers (NAPGCM)
655 N. Alvernon Way, Suite 108
Tucson, AZ 85711
(602) 881-8008

Promotes quality services and care for elderly citizens. Provides referral service and distributes information to individuals interested in geriatric care centers. Operates speakers' bureau; maintains referral network.

Publications: *Geriatric Care Manager*, quarterly.

HANDICAP

Clearinghouse on the Handicapped
Sweitzer Building, Room 3132
330 Cancer Street SW
Washington, DC 20202
(202) 732-1244

Responds to inquiries by referral to organizations that supply information to handicapped individuals relating to their own disabilities. Provides information on federal benefits, funding, and legislation.

OCCUPATIONAL SAFETY

National Safe Workplace Institute (NSWI)
5018 Park Rd.
Box 100
Charlotte, NC 28209
(704) 521-1212

Provides research and education on issues related to occupational health and safety. Concerned with safe and healthy work environments; seeks to make workplace safety and health a priority. Monitors efforts of the public and private sectors in improving workplace safety including the performance and activities of the U.S. Occupational Safety and Health Administration.

Publications: *Basic Information on Workplace Safety and Health in the U.S.*, annually.

National Safety Council (NSC)
1121 Spring Lake Dr.
Itasca, IL 60143-3201
(708) 285-1121

A voluntary nongovernmental organization. Promotes accident reduction by providing a forum for the exchange of safety and health ideas, techniques, and experiences and the discussion of accident prevention methods. Offers background courses at Safety Training Institute and home study courses for supervisors. Maintains extensive library on health and safety subjects.

Publications: *Accident Facts. Automotive, Tooling, Meatlworking and Associated Industries Newsletter*, bimonthly. *Family Safety and Health*, quarterly magazine. *Health Care Newsletter*, bimonthly. *Safety and Health*, monthly magazine. Covers all aspects of occupational safety and health.

School and Community Safety Society of America (SCSSA)
1900 Association Dr.
Reston, VA 22091
(703) 476-3430

Teachers and others professionally involved in the educational aspects of areas such as traffic safety education; emergency preparedness; health education for injury control; safety program management; professional preparation in safety; athletics, physical education and recreational sports safety; school/community/senior citizen/handicapped safety programming. Encourages the development of safety concepts and behaviors among its members.

Publications: *Safety Forum*, 2-3 times per year newsletter.

ORTHOPEDICS

American Academy of Orthopaedic Surgeons (AAOS)
6300 N. River Rd
Rosemont, IL 60018-4226
(708) 823-7186
(800)346-AAOS

Professional society of orthopedic surgeons certified by the American Board of Orthopedic Surgery to practice orthopedic (bone and joint) surgery.

Publications: *Bulletin*, quarterly.

American Association of Orthopedic Medicine (AAOM)
5147 Lewiston Rd.
Lewiston, NY 14092-1956
(716) 284-5777

Physicians and allied health professionals interested in the advancement of knowledge, diagnosis, and nonsurgical treatment of musculoskeletal and related disorders. Seeks to advance the standards of practice and quality of service in the field of orthopedic medicine; serves as a forum of learning for all of the specialties that deal with pain and dysfunction in the neural, muscular, skeletal, and vascular systems.

Publications: *AAOM Membership Directory*, annually. *AAOM News*, quarterly. *The Journal of Orthopaedic Medicine*, 3 times a year.

American Orthopaedic Foot and Ankle Society (AOFAS)
701 16th Ave.
Seattle, WA 98122
(800) 235-4855

Members of American Academy of Orthopaedic Surgeons interested in research on, education in, and care of the foot and ankle. Sponsors continuing medical education courses.

Publications: *The Adult Foot*, pamphlet. *The Child's* Foot, pamphlet. *In-Stride*, quarterly. Newsletter. *Journal of the Foot and Ankle*, bimonthly.

ORTHOTICS AND PROSTHETICS

American Academy of Orthotists and Prosthetists (AAOP)
1650 King St. Suite 500
Alexandria, VA 22314
(703) 836-7118

Certified professional practitioners in orthotics and prosthetics. Is dedicated to the advancement of the profession and the improvement of patient care. Conducts scientific seminars designed to increase professional competence of the individual practitioner.

Publications: *Academy Focus*, quarterly newsletter. Handbooks. *Journal of Prosthetics and Orthotics*, quarterly. Manuals. Also publishes audiovisual equipment.

American Orthotic and Prosthetic Association
1650 Kings St., Suite 500
Alexandria, VA 22314
(703) 836-7116

Firms that manufacture and fit artificial braces.

Publications: *Almanac*, monthly. *Journal of Prosthetics*, quarterly.

Association of Children's Prosthetic-Orthotic Clinics (ACPOC)
6300 N. River Rd., No. 727
Rosemont, IL 60018
(708) 698-1694

Prosthetic-orthotic clinics for children. Promotes the exchange of information concerning children's prosthetic-orthotic devices. Fosters cooperative research development and evaluative efforts among member clinics. Seeks to improve care in member clinics.

Publications: *Journal of the Association of Children's Prosthetic-Orthotic Clinics*, quarterly.

PEDIATRICS

American Academy of Pediatrics (AAP)
141 Northwest Point Blvd.
P.O. Box 927
Elk Grove, IL 60009-0927
(708) 228-5005

Professional medical society of pediatricians and pediatric specialists. Operates small member library of books and journals on pediatric medicine, office practice, and child health care policy. Maintains 42 committees, councils, and tasks forces including: Accident and Poison Prevention;

Publications: *AAP NEWS*, monthly. *Fellowship List*, annually. *Pediatrics*, monthly journal. *Pediatrics in Review*, monthly journal.

PHYSICAL THERAPY

American Physical Therapy Association (APTA)
111 N. Fairfax St.
Alexandria, VA 22314
(703) 684-2782

Professional organization of physical therapists and physical therapist assistants and students. Fosters the development and improvement of physical therapy service; directs the maintenance standards and promotes scientific research. Offers advisory and consultation services to schools of physical therapy and facilities offering physical therapy services.

Publications: Brochures. Monographs, *Physical Therapy*, monthly journal. *PT Bulletin*, weekly newsletter. *PT Magazine*, monthly journal. *Today's Student in PT*, semi-annual.

Orthopaedic Section, American Physical Therapy Association
505 King St., Suite 103
La Crosse, WI 54601
(608) 784-0910
(800) 444-3982

Supports the continued growth of the physical therapy profession through education and research; promotes development of a standard certification procedure for the field. Seeks to assure the quality of physical therapy curricula at both the undergraduate and postgraduate levels. Facilitates communication among orthopedic physical therapists and other health care professionals. Gathers and disseminates information on the care of musculoskeletal disorders.

Publications: Brochure. *Journal of Orthopaedic and Sports Physical Therapy*, monthly. *Orthopaedic Physical Therapy Practice*, quarterly.

PODIATRY

American College of Foot and Ankle Surgeons (ACFAS)
444 N. Northwest Hwy., Suite 150
Park Ridge, IL 60068
(708) 292-2237

Objectives are to promote and disseminate information on podiatric surgery; encourage and publish research findings and related literature.

Publications: *American College of Foot and Ankle Surgeons*, quarterly newsletter. *Complications in Foot and Ankle Surgery*. *Journal of Foot and Ankle Surgery*, quarterly.

REFLEX SYMPATHETIC DYSTROPHY

Lupus Foundation of America (LFA)
4 Research Place, Suite 180
Rockville, MD 20850-3226
(301) 670-9292
(800) 558-0121

Nonprofit voluntary health foundation serving people with lupus erythematosus and their families. Objectives are to provide patient education, services, and human support to members; educate the medical community and the public about the disease in order to obtain earlier diagnoses and better treatment for lupus patients.

Publications: *Lupus Erythematosus: A Handbook for Physicians, Patients and their Families* (in English and Spanish). *Lupus News*, 3 times per year newsletter. *Understanding Lupus*.

Lupus Network (LN)
230 Ranch Dr.
Bridgeport, CT 06606
(203) 372-5795

Educators, medical professionals, and individuals suffering from systemic lupus erythematosus. Seeks to foster better understanding of the disease among patients, educators, and professionals through the distribution of educational materials.

Publications: Brochures. *Heliogram*, quarterly newsletter.

Reflex Sympathetic Dystrophy Association (RSDSA)
P.O. Box 821
Haddonfield, NJ 08033
(609) 795-8845

People with Reflex Sympathetic Dystrophy Syndrome; health care professional treating RSDS patients. Conducts media campaigns; encourages and supports RSDS treatment and research; has a national data bank for the coordination of RSDS research and treatment information. Aid in the formation of support groups for people with RSDS; makes available referral services. Conducts educational programs; maintains speakers' bureau; compiles statistics.

Publications: *Help Us to Stop the Pain*, brochure. Newsletter, quarterly. *RSDS Digest*, annually.

The American Lupus Society (TALS)
3914 Del Amo Blvd, Suite 922
Torrance, CA 90503
(310) 542-8891
(800) 331-1802

Works to increase knowledge and public awareness of lupus erythematosus, a noncontagious disease which may affect the skin alone or may manifest itself as a chronic, systemic, and inflammatory disease of the connective tissues. Assists lupus patients and their families, through chapters and patient support groups, to cope with the daily problems associated with lupus. Collects and distributes funds for research.

Publications: *The American Lupus Society - Lupus Today*, quarterly newsletter. Booklet, for children. *Lupus Erythematosus*, pamphlet. Also publishes other informational materials in Braile and Spanish.

RETIREMENT

American Association of Retired Persons (AARP)
601 E. St. NW
Washington, DC 20049
(202) 434-2277

Persons 50 years of age or older, working or retired. Seeks to improve every aspect of living for older people. Has targeted four areas of immediate concern: health care, women's initiative, worker equity, and minority affairs. Provides group health insurance program, discounts on auto rental and hotel rates, and a specially designed and priced motoring plan. Sponsors community service programs on crime prevention, defensive driving, and tax aid, and the AARP Andrus Foundation, which awards grants to universities for gerontology research. Provides pre-retirement planning program; offers special services to retired teachers through National Retired Teachers Association, Division of AARP. Sponsors mail order pharmacy services.

Publications: *AARP News Bulletin*, 11 times per year newsletter. *Modern Maturity*, bimonthly magazine. *Working Age*, bimonthly newsletter. Also publishes books on housing, health, exercise, retirement planning, money management, and travel and leisure.

Association of Retired Americans (ARA)
9102 N. Meridan St., Suite 405
Indianapolis, IN 46260
(317) 571-6888

Senior Americans intersted in enhancing their lives through group benefits. Purpose is to offer a program of high quality, low-cost benefits and services to members. Services available through ARA are discounts on prescription, eyeglasses, and hearing aids; low interest credit cards; discounts on lodging, car rental, tours, cruises, and airfare; insurance benefits including emergency air medical transportation. Assists governmental bodies and agencies with the development of programs and legislation which benefit and promote the well-being of retired Americans.

Publications: *Vintage Times*, quarterly.

RHEUMATIC DISEASES

American Juvenile Arthritis Organization (AJAO)
1314 Spring St. NW
Atlanta, GA 30309
(404) 872-7100

Parents, health care professional and others interested in the problems of juvenile arthritis. Advocates for the needs of those affected by juvenile arthritis. A council of the Arthritis Foundation.

Publications: *AJAO Newsletter*, quarterly. *Arthritis in Children*, brochure. *Educational Rights for Children with Arthritis: A Manual for Parents. Juvenile Dermatomyositis, When Your Student has Arthritis*, brochure.

Arthritis Foundation (AF)
1314 Spring St. NW
Atlanta, GA 30309
(404) 872-7100
(800) 283-7800

Seeks to discover the cause and improve the methods for the treatment and prevention of arthritis and other rheumatic diseases; increase the number of scientists investigating rheumatic diseases; extend knowledge of arthritis and other rheumatic diseases to the lay public, emphasizing the socioeconomic as well as medical aspects of these diseases.

Publications: *Arthritis Today*, bimonthly magazine. *Bulletin on the Rheumatic Diseases*, bimonthly.

Arthritis Health Professions Association (AHPA)
1314 Spring St. NW
Atlanta, GA 30309
(404) 872-7100

Nurses, occupational and physical therapists, social workers, psychologists, vocational counselors, physicians, pharmacists, and other health professionals concerned with the practice, education, and research of rheumatic diseases. Disseminates information regarding the study and treatment of rheumatic diseases. Develops and implements medical and scientific programs in the field of rheumatology. A section of the Arthritis Foundation.

Publications: *Arthritis Care and Research*, quarterly. *Arthritis Today*, quarterly. *Bulletin on the Rheumatic Diseases*, 12 times a year. *Guide to Independent*

Living for People with Arthritis. Newsletter, periodic. *Outcome Standards for Rheumatology Nursing Practice. Primer on the Rheumatic Diseases.*

National Arthritis and Musculoskeletal and Skin Diseases Information Clearinghouse (NAMSIC)
9000 Rockville Pile
P.O Box AMS
Bethesda, MD 20892-2903
(301) 495-4484

Collects, publishes, and disseminates professional and public educational materials for persons concerned with arthritis and musculoskeletal and skin diseases.

Publications: *Arthritis, Rheumatic Diseases, and Related Disorders*, annual report. *Spanish Language Materials for Patients: a Bibliography on Arthritis, Musculoskeletal and Skin Diseases* (In Spanish).

SPORTS MEDICINE

American College of Sports Medicine (ACSM)
P.O. Box 1440
Indianapolis, IN 46206-1440
(317) 637-9200

Promotes the integration of scientific research and practical applications of sports medicine and exercise science to maintains and enhance physical performance, fitness, health, and quality of life. Certifies fitness leaders, fitness instructors, exercise test technologists, exercise specialists, health/fitness program directors, and U.S. military fitness personnel.

Publications: *ACSM Fitness Book. ACSM's Health/Fitness Facility Standards and Guidelines. American College of Sports Medicine Career Services Bulletin*, monthly newsletter. Lists career and fellowship opportunities in sports medicine in the U.S. and aboard. *American College of Sports Medicine Directory of Graduate Programs in Sports Medicine and Exercise Science*, annual. Lists graduate programs in fields related to exercise science and sports medicine at North American institutions. *Medicine and Science in Sports and Exercise* , monthly journal. *Sports Medicine Bulletin*, quarterly newsletters.

American Orthopaedic Society for Sports Medicine (AOSSM)
6300 N. River Rd., Suite 200
Rosemont, IL 60018
(708) 292-4900

Orthopedic surgeons working in sports medicine; others in related fields involved in the care of athletes. Increases the knowledge and improves care of athletic injuries. Performs educational and research functions; disseminates information.

Publications: *American Journal of Sports Medicine*, bimonthly. Reports on the diagnosis, treatment, prevention, and rehabilitation of sports-related injury and disease; also includes society news and book reviews.

Index